Journey Through Menopause

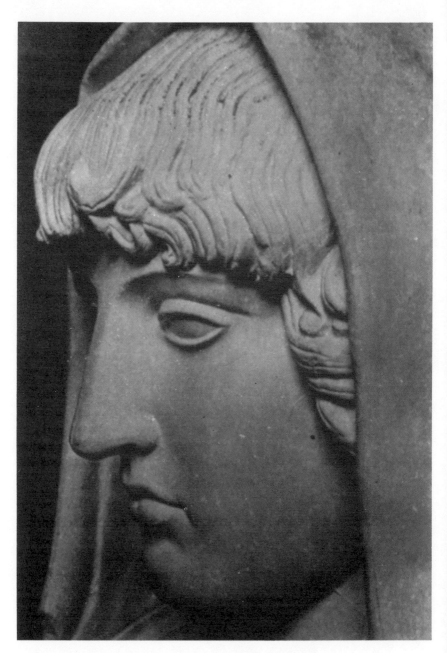

1. Hestia Giustiniani, marble, 5th c. B.C.E., Villa Albani, Rome.

JOURNEY THROUGH MENOPAUSE

A Personal Rite of Passage

Christine Downing

CROSSROAD • NEW YORK

1987

The Crossroad Publishing Company
370 Lexington Avenue, New York, N.Y. 10017

Printed in the United States of America

Library of Congress Cataloging in Publication Data

Downing, Christine, 1931–
    Journey through menopause.

    1. Menopause — Psychological aspects.   2. Menopause —
Social aspects.   3. Downing, Christine, 1931–   Health.
4. Women — United States — Biography.   I. Title.
RG186.D68   1987   612'.665   87–8994
ISBN 0-8245-0836-X

For Tom and for River

Affairs are now soul size
— Christopher Fry

CONTENTS

ILLUSTRATIONS

ACKNOWLEDGMENTS

I want to thank

Eleanor Garner for telling me upon first reading "Come and Celebrate With Me": this should be a book.

Richard Underwood for dreaming with me of a different book than the one which has come into being, a book which would have included *his* journey through the midlife passage.

Elaine Estwick for keeping the letters I wrote from my trip around the world.

Janet Gunn for her trust that the stories about my trip around the world had meaning for others.

Melvin and *Beth Keiser* for the conversation during which the shape for this book came into focus.

George Lawler, whose dissatisfaction with the first version of the book led me to rework it.

Frank Oveis, my editor at Crossroad, whose appreciation of the book renewed my own.

Janet Hamann and *Elaine Estwick* for typing and retyping.

Clare Oksnër, Lilla Sweatt, and *Grace Mann* for helping me find the illustrations.

Thomas Hollander for traveling with me.

River Malcolm for living with me.

Earlier versions of "Come and Celebrate With Me" appeared in *WomanSpirit* and in *Anima*, of "Coming Home to Hestia" in *Lady Unique*. Work on this project was supported in part by grants from the National Endowment for the Humanities and the San Diego State University Foundation.

Christine Downing
Del Mar, California

I
PREAMBLE

FEMALE RITES
OF PASSAGE

*Men, once initiated, never get the
second chance. They never change
again. That's their loss, not ours.
Why borrow poverty?*
— *Ursula LeGuin*

On my fiftieth birthday I realized: if I live to be as old as my mother already is, I am now just beginning the second half of my adult life. I knew myself to be at the point of transition from early to late adulthood. I knew that because I am a woman this turning would be definitively marked by the physiological phenomenon of menopause. I suspected that the social, psychological, and spiritual dimensions of my experiencing this life-change were all likely to be so affected by the biological event as to make what had been written about mid-life crisis by men (for whom aging is a continuous process) seem mostly beside the point. Yet I knew almost nothing of the distinctively female ways of navigating this passage and felt myself to be confronting a transition for which my culture had somehow conspired to keep me unprepared. I felt alone, uninformed, somewhat afraid — and yet also curious and expectant. I was at the brink of a centrally important life-change and had no knowledge of the myths or rituals that had helped women throughout history live this transition with hope, dignity, and depth.

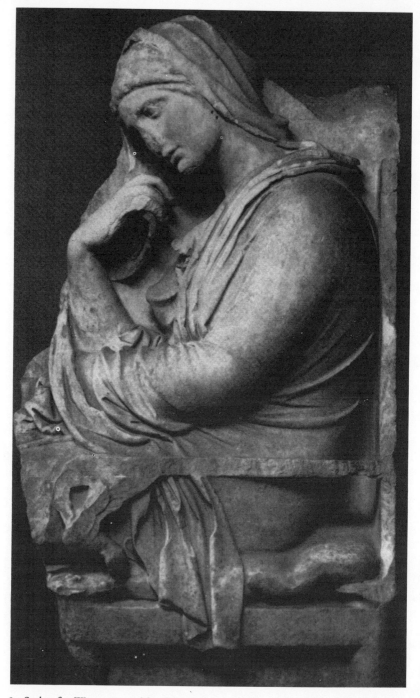

2. Stele of a Woman, marble, 4th c. B.C.E., Attica, Metropolitan Museum, New York.

I knew that from the day of birth to that of death individuals in traditional cultures submit to ceremonies which make possible the passage from one social category or life phase to another. Sometimes individuals have to undergo the transition alone; sometimes they are led through it in the company of other members of a particular group within the society. As Arnold Van Gennep noted in his classical study, *Les rites des passage*, published some seventy-five years ago, participation in such ritualized passages was regarded as an ineluctable feature of human life:

> For groups, as well as for individuals, life itself means to separate and to be reunited, to change form and condition, to die and be reborn. It is to act and to cease, to wait and rest, and then to begin acting again, but in a different way. And there are always new thresholds to cross: the thresholds of summer and winter, of a season or a year, of a month or a night; the thresholds of birth, adolescence, maturity, and old age; the threshold of death and that of the afterlife — for those who believe in it . . .
>
> The series of human transitions has, among some peoples, been linked to the celestial passages, the revolutions of the planets, and the phases of the moon. It is indeed a cosmic conception that relates the stages of human existence to those of plant and animal life and, by a sort of pre-scientific divination, joins them to the great rhythms of the universe.[1]

Rites of passage serve to reveal the social significance of what might otherwise appear as individual crises (puberty, childbirth, illness, journeys, death); their purpose is to integrate the personal and the transpersonal. Through participation in such rites one discovers that one's suffering and confusion are not unique and isolating. The pain one endures in giving up and leaving behind a familiar and cherished life form is simply the pain of being human, what Freud calls "common unhappiness." Because the ritual was communal, participation in it provides validation that, having passed through the initiatory experience, one is truly a new person. One is not only different to oneself, one is met by others as being different. Participation in a sequence of such rites which have always the same form—separation, initiation, reincorporation—leads one toward an appreciation of the rhythms of life and gives meaning to the transition time as going somewhere, as not a cul-de-sac or dead end. The rites are often supplemented by myths which recount how a prototypical goddess or god, heroine or hero, was the first to undergo the same trial and to discover its hidden significance. The rituals and myths serve to alleviate the potentially harmful effects of significant life transitions on the affected individuals and their communities.

Although in modern societies there are few such explicit transitional rituals, the initiatory pattern may still continue to function, albeit unconsciously, in our imaginative and dream life and in certain real challenges we undergo. Mircea Eliade believes the pattern to be visible "in the spiritual crises, the solitude and despair through which every human being must pass in order to attain to a responsible, genuine and creative life":

> Even if the initiatory character of these ordeals is not apprehended, as such, nevertheless it remains true that humans become themselves only after having solved a series of desperately difficult and even dangerous situations; that is, after having undergone "tortures" and "death," followed by an awakening to another life, qualitatively different because regenerated. If we look closely, we see that every human life is made up of a series of ordeals, of "deaths," and of "resurrections.". . . Initiation lies at the core of any genuine human life.[2]

Eliade speaks to those of us who feel a persistent longing for a more conscious relation to the archetypal pattern, and for shared rituals and myths to help us through our most significant trials and transitions. The symbols might help assuage the loneliness of experiencing the difficulties of our passages as idiosyncratic, the terror of experiencing them as pathological, the despair of not finding in them any symbolical or analogical meaning.

The hope that awareness of how others in our culture commonly live through the transitions from one life phase to the next would provide us with some of the cultural wisdom and collective support formerly given by rite and myth may help account for the popularity of such books as Gail Sheehy's *Passages* and Dan Levinson's *Seasons of a Man's Life*. Both move beyond the fetishistic focus on puberty rites which has helped obscure what we all really know: that there are initiations beyond those associated with adolescence that are difficult and lonely, particularly the mid-life entrance into late adulthood.

That our lives, as surely as the primitive's, proceed through a typical series of crises, critical steps, and turning points is the central premise underlying Erik Erikson's charting of "the eight ages of man." His typology assumes:

> (1) that the human personality in principle develops according to steps predetermined in the growing person's readiness to be driven toward, to be aware of, and to interact with, a widening social radius; and (2) that society, in principle, tends to be so constituted as to meet and invite this succession of potentialities for interaction and attempts to safeguard and to encourage the proper rate and proper sequence of their unfolding. This is the "maintenance of the human world."[3]

Perhaps because his stages were originally conceived as part of a study of childhood, the emphasis is so much on early life transitions that only the last two pertain to adulthood. In early adulthood, as Erikson describes it, the conflict is between generativity and stagnation, the task is that of meeting one's responsibilities to the community, particularly to the next generation. The characteristic task of the last stage, late adulthood, the balancing of "ego integrity vs. despair," ideally issues in "renunciation and wisdom," in a post-narcissistic acceptance of one's particular life story and of one's inescapable death. But Erikson's delineation of these adult stages is little more than a sketch and he has nothing to say of wht happens when society fails adequately to invite or meet transitions which are nevertheless forced upon us. He takes no account of the conspiracy of silence Simone de Beauvoir saw to surround the status of being old (or "coming of age") in our culture. His perfunctoriness seems to confirm Proust's conviction that aging "of all realities is perhaps that of which we retain a purely abstract notion longest in our lives."[4]

Few of us share Jan Rule's aspiration:

> To become an old woman has always been my ambition. . . .
> As my grandmothers taught me the real lessons of erotic
> love with their beautifully requiring flesh and speaking
> faces, so I would wish to teach the children I love that they
> are capable of tenderness and strength, capable of knowl-
> edge because of what they can see in my face, clear in pain
> and wonder, intent on practicing life as long as it lasts.[5]

For most of us old age is always something that begins later, further down the pike. Because we regard the elderly as radically *other*, we seem to view them always only from outside. Thus aging is seen as without subjective, existential, psychological significance.

Yet fifty years ago Carl Jung was already insisting on the intrinsic meaning of what he called "the second half of life":

A human being would certainly not grow to be seventy or eighty years old if this longevity had no meaning for the species. The afternoon of human life must also have a significance of its own and cannot be merely a pitiful appendage to life's morning.[6]

Jung saw this significance as having to do with life's afternoon being a time for attention to the inward rather than the outward world, for attention to symbolic rather than literal meaning. That he knew the shift in orientation may be confusing and painful is powerfully documented by the account of the trauma of his own mid-life crisis presented in the "Confrontation with the Unconscious" chapter of his autobiography.[7] Having negotiated the passage, he came to see his own therapeutic gifts as particularly adapted to helping others experience the transition into the second half of life as soul event.

Jung, however, had no particular interest in the specific ways in which women may experience the mid-life passage (perhaps in part because of his tendency to disregard those correlations between physiological and psychological change so much emphasized by Freud). In this neglect he was, of course, simply repeating with respect to contemporary life what has long been true of anthropological explorations of traditional cultures. As Eliade observes, female initiations have in general been much less studied than male, because such rites, especially in their secret aspects, have been less accessible to (primarily male) ethnologists. Eliade nevertheless believes it to be established that girls' puberty initiations are less widespread than those of boys, less intricately developed and more individual. The last characteristic he attributes to the fact that female initiation begins with the first menstruation; the physical symptom is directly understood as a symbol of sexual maturity and leads to immediate social recognition in the form of isolation.[8] Since the transition has a directly physiological correlate, it is not simply conventional, social, as is the boy's assumption of adulthood. Because the girl's transformation is less diffuse, it may need less explicit ceremonial delineation.

Yet Eliade acknowledges that girls are often brought together into groups where they are taught the secrets of sexuality and fertility. The teaching is in essence religious: "It consists in a revelation of the sacrality of women. The girl is ritually prepared to assume her specific mode of being, that is, to become a creatress." At the same time she is taught "her responsibilities in society and in the cosmos, responsibilities which, among primitives, are always religious in nature." Eliade speaks of how among many peoples female initiation takes place in several stages: what begins with the first menses is elaborated during the first pregnancy and completed with the birth of the first child.

> Girls' initiations are determined by a mystery "natural" to the female sex, the appearance of menstruation, with all this phenomenon implies for primitives: e.g., periodical purification, fecundity, curative and magical powers. The girl is to become conscious of a transformation that comes about in a natural way and to assume the mode of being that results from it, the mode of being of the adult woman. . . . For girls, initiation involves a series of revelations concerning the secret meaning of a phenomenon that is apparently natural—the visible sign of their sexual maturity.[9]

Eliade is explicitly cognizant of the specificity of female religious experience, of the existence of two different modes of sacrality—masculine and feminine. He implies that female initiation is an initiation into the natural rhythms of life (rather than a forced induction into culture viewed as opposed to nature), and that the focus is not so much on the undergoing of ordeals as on the acceptance of a given change.[10]

In recent years, in large measure in response to the contemporary women's movement, we have begun to know much more than Eliade did when he wrote *Rites and Symbols of Initiation* about the details and variety of female religiosity and rituals.[11] We are beginning to learn more not just about the outwardly visible cultic behavior but, even more importantly, about the *meaning* of this behavior to the female participants. Our own experience of menarche and of motherhood has been deepened as we have learned how these female mysteries were celebrated in the myths and rituals of other cultures. However, we have no comparable evidence for the traditional understanding of menopause. What Van Gennep said still seems to be true: "There do not seem to be any rites of menopause." Nor, he went on to say,

> of the greying of hair, though these both mark the beginning of a new phase of life which is very important among the semicivilized. In general, either old women become identified with the men and therefore participate in their ceremonies, political activities and so forth, or they acquire a special position within their own sex group, especially as ceremonial leaders.[12]

De Beauvoir agrees: "Neither for men nor for women do we anywhere find initiation ceremonies that confirm the status of being an elder."[13]

I long for relevant myths and rites but find there are almost none, perhaps because in primitive cultures so few women live long enough to reach menopause. Although I am glad to know that there are important rituals and sacred roles reserved to postmenopausal women in traditional societies where age is venerated more than it is in ours, I still wish for rituals associated with the passage itself. That unappeased longing has led me to believe that we must create our own rites of separation and passage by beginning to tell one another not only about the physical aspects of our experience of menopause but also about our dreams and nightmares, our fears, our hopes, our strange fantasies and unwilled wishes. I recall how spontaneously my fifth and sixth grade classmates and I created our own ritualization of puberty as we shared our questions and fantasies about sexuality and our stories about our first periods. I remember also the hours I spent as a young mother with my women friends telling one another about our pregnancies and our deliveries. Now I want to know how my experience of menopause relates to that of others, my mother, my grandmother, my sister, my friends, women everywhere.

That the rituals of separation from an outworn phase of life are ones that we must create for ourselves is intimated in Adrienne Rich's poem, "Toward the Solstice":

> If some rite of separation
> is still unaccomplished
> between myself and the long-gone
> tenants of this house,
> between myself and my childhood,
> and the childhood of my children,
> it is I who have neglected
> to perform the needed acts,
> set water in corners, light and eucalyptus
> in front of mirrors,
> or merely pause and listen
> to my own pulse vibrating
> lightly as falling snow,
> relentlessly as the rainstorm,
> and hear what it has been saying.
> It seems I am still waiting

for them to make some clear demand
some articulate sound or gesture,
for release to come from anywhere
but from inside myself.[14]

It makes me sad to know that if someone speaks of the myths of menstruation or menopause, they mean the untruths, the fallacies, the misogynist distortions. I cannot believe that I am alone in my hunger for a more symbolic connection to these mysteries of feminine life. Our relation to these profoundly life-transforming transitions (and thus to ourselves and to our sisters) seems so obviously diminished when we live them as though they don't really matter very much, when we experience them as degrading, as isolating and isolated events, as taboo.

I understand why some have called for a demythologizing of menopause[15] — that is, for its dissociation from a long-familiar congeries of coincidentally or subjectively associated phenomena — but what I believe we really require is a *remythologizing* of it. I would wish us to learn to view menopause developmentally rather than pathologically, as a life phase rather than a degenerative or deficiency disease, and to see it not only as a physiological event but as a psychological one, as a soul experience.

I had hoped that Esther Harding (whose *Woman's Mysteries* so profoundly explores the relevance of ancient mythological traditions to the self-understanding of contemporary women) would have some wisdom to offer about the soul dimension of the menopausal passage. But when I read the chapter called "Autumn and Winter" in her *The Way of All Women*, I was disappointed that she referred to menopause in only one casual phrase ("the loss of her moon-cycle"). I was also puzzled that she seemed to differentiate hardly at all between "autumn" and "winter."[16] Even Jung had known enough to distinguish clearly between "afternoon" and "evening." Surely the experience and tasks of a fifty-year-old woman like myself differ radically from that of an eighty-year-old like my mother. Yet I began to wonder if Harding's failure to emphasize the differences might not be rooted in an implicit recognition that the lives of women may be more easily understood in terms of three seasons than of four and that the pattern of climactic descent at mid-life may pertain more to male than female experience. The threefold cycle of the initiation process — birth, life, death; separation, initiation, return; conception, growth, emergence — has always seemed to me the most appropriate description of the life process, as it also did to the ancient Greeks. Their mythology included three Horae, three seasons: Thallo, Karpo, and Auxo — growth, flowering, ripeness. To express her relation to all the phases of female life, they represented the goddess, Hera, in three aspects: as Hera Parthenos, Hera Teleia, and Hera Chera — as maiden, wife, and post-connubial woman. Persephone's life, too, is divided into thirds and Hekate, the goddess of crossroads and transitions, is known as three-faced Hekate. The underworld (which is for Greeks the realm of the soul) is ruled by the Eleusinian triad — maiden, mother, and crone. There are, it now seems obvious, three seasons to a woman's life, irrespective of whether she is heterosexual, homosexual, or celibate, quite apart from whether she has ever conceived or borne or nursed a child: from birth to menarche, menarche to menopause, menopause to death (and within each a threefold initiatory structure as well).

It is my conviction that the phases of a woman's life are different from those of a man's and that the female mid-life transition is different from the male. Because for women the transition is inevitably associated with the physiological marker, menopause, it is apt to come somewhat later, more likely at fifty than at forty. Rather than suddenly coming upon us, it seems to be naturally connected to our own internal rhythms. It may involve less in the way of radical reversal than often seems true for men. Certainly the image of having at mid-life to kill and then bury an old self, which Murray Stein finds central to the male transition, is too violent, too dramatic, to express my own experience. It seems odd that the social experience of external mid-life readjustments and the biological experience of menstrual termination are treated so separately in most published accounts of contemporary women's own explorations—and odder still how little the inner psychical aspect is considered at all. (Lillian Rubin's *Women of a Certain Age: The Midlife Search for Self*, for example, doesn't even include "menopause" in its index.) The medical research suggests that for most women (as was true for me) the only physical indicators explicitly associated with menopause (and not with aging per se) are hot flashes, and that only a small proportion of women who experience such flashes find them troubling. Nevertheless the most distinguishing characteristic of menopause from a medical perspective seems to be the likelihood that some therapeutic measures are being employed! In our culture, especially among middle-class Caucasians, a majority of women are given tranquilizers or estrogen and a high proportion some gynecological surgery, often despite the lack of specific symptoms necessitating these measures.[17] I suspect that viewing the physical signs as symptoms in need of medical treatment is yet another domain in which the meaning of female experience has been defined by males. I cannot help but wonder if it might not be some other form of *therapeia* (attention of the kind one gives the sacred) that is really required. Understanding menopause as primarily a physical experience may block access to its spiritual significance.

I am persuaded that it is time for us to begin telling one another of our inner experience of menopause. I think of the power of Audre Lorde's testimony in *The Cancer Journals* of the importance of our talking to one another about taboo experiences:

> For other women of all ages, colors, and sexual identities
> who recognize that imposed silence about any area of our
> lives is a tool for separation and powerlessness, and for my-
> self, I have tried to voice some of my feelings and thoughts
> about the travesty of prothesis, the pain of amputation, the
> function of cancer in a profit economy, my confrontation
> with mortality, the strength of women loving, and the
> power and rewards of self-conscious living.[18]

I, too, would like to speak of how it has been for me in a way
that would be of service to other women. Thus, I have written
this book as an account of my journey through menopause, in
the hope that it will initiate a new openness among us about this
area of our lives.

My experience is inevitably to some degree idiosyncratic. It is
part of the cost of the imposed silence that I cannot know how
much of it is typical or how much of it will be illuminating to
others as they prepare themselves for a passage still before them
or as they seek to understand more profoundly the meaning of a
passage already taken. My journey took place over a three year
period and followed the typical pattern of the rite of passage:
preparation, transition, and return. The preparatory phase was
initiated by a dream which announced that it was time for me to
make ready and which thus sent me to examining what psychology, mythology, and my own dreams could tell me about
the transition I was about to undergo. The task of writing "Come
and Celebrate with Me" was itself a work of purification and the
beginning of my separation from the assumptions and attachments of my premenopausal self. Dreams were for me the primary vehicle of preparation.

A year later I found myself undertaking a journey around the
world which turned out to be my literal passage through menopause. Van Gennep had written that traditionally the passage

from one social position to another is identified with a *territorial* passage:

> This identification explains why the passage from one group to another is so often ritually expressed by passage under a portal, or by an "opening of doors." These phrases and events are seldom meant as "symbols"; for the semi-civilized the passage is actually a territorial passage.[19]

I had not forseen this would be true for me. Yet the journeying did serve to emphasize the ritual aspect of the transition. The trip functioned as a publicly visible event which insured that others would know I was returning as a different person. My preparations seemed in large measure irrelevant, except that they had opened me to live the menopausal transition consciously and symbolically. Where I had hoped to have communion, I found myself undertaking a radically solitary journey; where I had expected to be immersed in feminine reality, I found myself engaged in a struggle with the masculine; where I had anticipated being taught by dream and myth, I found myself learning from strangers, events, and landscapes met in an outer though utterly unfamiliar world. I would not expect that others would embark on a similar voyage but do believe that my journey brought into view in magnified form the motifs and challenges that belong to the "normal" experience of menopause — much as psychopathology in its exaggerations reveals the structure of normal consciousness. The whole trip was like a myth or highly elaborated dream. It took me out of the everyday world and everyday temporality into liminal spatiality, a sacred arena where each person, place, and incident was charged with meaning. That attunement to the soul dimension of this worldly event may in itself have been the most important lesson of the journey. Menopause initiates one into a time of life when symbolic consciousness is appropriately part of everyday experience—at home as well as on the road, in waking life and not only in dream. But there were other lessons also: the discovery that I was at last done with the heroic quest, the acceptance of physical weakness and vulnerability, the recognition of my dependence on other women; the revelation that I am loved enough.

The journey brought me home, and at home I found myself a postmenopausal woman engaged in the tasks of the reincorporation phase: assimilation, integration, and finding a way to share what I had experienced. I found myself in tutelage to a divinity not even considered in the preparatory phase: Hestia, the Greek goddess of hearth and home. I found myself not in quest of home but: home. For the first time I felt I truly understood the sacredness inherent in the simple fact of being home.

Yet having completed my journey through menopause, I know myself to be standing at the beginning of another life-stage. From the day of birth to that of death. . . .

II
THE PREPARATION

COME AND CELEBRATE
WITH ME

Now that I am fifty-six
Come and celebrate with me —

What happens to song and sex
Now that I am fifty-six?

They dance, but differently,
Death and distance in the mix;
Now that I am fifty-six
Come and celebrate with me.
                    — Muriel Rukeyser

S hortly before my fiftieth birthday I had a dream in which my former husband and I were walking among steeply sloping sand dunes like those I remember from my childhood. From time to time we could see the ocean, waves breaking high. The wind was blowing enough to make talking difficult; the dune grass cut into our calves; the sand shifted underfoot. We were intent on our walking, giving one another a hand now and then at a particularly tricky spot, thoroughly enjoying being together. At some point along the way, when we had slowed our pace a bit, I said, "You know, dear, I think I'm pregnant again, and this time I don't even know who the father is."

"Will we keep it?" he asked.

"We always do, don't we?" I replied.

21

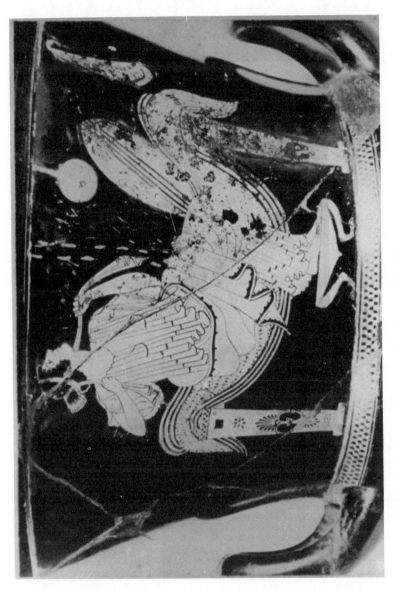

3. Conception of the Divine Child. Danaë and the Shower of Gold, terracotta, 5th c. B.C.E., Attica, The Hermitage, Leningrad.

When I awoke, I asked, as one would, "Now where did that come from?" I realized that without having particularly noticed it, I had gone several weeks beyond the time when I would ordinarily have begun to menstruate. In my dream life I was pregnant; in waking life I was probably experiencing the first signs of menopause.

But in waking life, too, I felt myself pregnant with something, my menopausal self, perhaps. The dream image needed to be attended to, not dismissed as a regressive, evasive fantasy nor severed from what was going on in my body. Sometimes women of nearly fifty do conceive; if I, too, were literally pregnant, then that would become evident soon enough. Meanwhile it felt important to live with the dream image, honoring its reality. I found I loved especially that this dreamchild would have no known father, would be entirely *my* child. One morning I awoke knowing her name: Melissa, a name I didn't particularly like and with which I had no conscious associations, but which was indubitably the dreamchild's name. I learned that to the Greeks Melissa was a bee whose honey induced madness and cured disease, was used in libations for the dead, and fed to infants to impart to them such numinous qualities as wisdom and eloquence. In Greek mythology Melissa was the first priestess of the great mother, the first human to sacrifice to the gods; priestesses of Demeter and Artemis were called by her name. That she was named after Melissa, the priestess who honors both Demeter, the goddess of motherhood, and Artemis, the goddess of self-sufficient womanhood, thus implied that my dreamchild was singularly well fitted to initiate me to the mysteries of menopause.

I missed another period and then began to flow at fairly regular intervals again. But the dream marked the beginning of my preparation for menopause.

It seemed appropriate to devote the Mother's Day weekend of my fiftieth year to trying to understand as best I could the soul meaning of the transition in which I was soon to be engaged, as several winters earlier at the time of my divorce I had given a weekend to Hera. I had wanted then to come to terms as wholly as I could—ritually and mythically, personally and archetypically—with all that wifehood had meant to me, as blessing and as curse, and all that leaving it behind would mean, as release and as loss. Now it was time for another such sorting through. Again I surrounded myself with books of poetry and myth, with dream journals and letters. I mused and scribbled, read and remembered, smiled and wept, saw and was mystified....

The setting was different. I began outside in the sun, surrounded by irises and roses; hummingbirds and butterflies were flitting nearby; a gentle breeze carried a bit of the ocean to me; the sky was a cloudless blue. It was a spring scene, as the scene of that other denouement had been a winter one. It felt like that, too, as though this transition would have more to do with beginnings than endings. But before I was done, I had moved inside, night had fallen. I had discovered again that to speak honestly meant truly honoring the darkness: fears, regrets, uncertainties. It meant attending to the dreams of dismemberment and death, not only to the dreams of pregnancy and rejuvenation with which I had innocently begun. Spring seems always to return me to the unsullied maidenly aspect of Persephone but menopause connects to darker dimensions of the Eleusian cult, to the dread goddess of the underworld and to her fearsome sister-self, Hekate, goddess of thresholds. Song and sex now dance with "death and distance in the mix."

At some level I must have known that all along, for I had almost immediately found myself remembering some other Mother's Days when images of death and birth had been confusedly intertwined: Mother's Day eve a decade earlier, marked by my oldest son's psychotic break, perhaps the first real "break" in my mothering and in that sense a prelude to menopause. Mother's

Day eve two years later, which began with a dream in which I received an invitation from this same son (long since recovered from his initiatory journey through madness) to the Magic Theater's performance of "Ego, Death, Process, Transformation," which ended with a night-long testing during which I was certain I was dying but was led instead to the discovery of "a center at the center" whose reality I had until then always doubted. A more recent Mother's Day, the first to be celebrated in this house between mountains and sea in which I hope to live for the rest of my years, a celebration which culminated in the conception of a child I knew from the beginning could only live imaginally. Even then, though menopause itself still lay several years ahead, I consciously experienced that conception as an initiation into a period of life when literal mothering had become beside the point.

This Mother's Day eve, while still immersed in my reflections about the meaning of menopause, my menstrual flow began—undeniable reminder that I was still in the preparatory phase of this transition. That bodily reminder called me back to my body and to an hour or more spent with and *as* the changing body that is me—seeing, touching, caressing. I realized then how important it is to me to speak of the body and from the body.

The weekend set aside as the beginning of my preparation for menopause led me to this passionate affirmation:

> I know menopause is not just a trivial little change whose rough spots can be eased with a little hormone treatment, on the other side of which I will still have a good figure and a good mind, still be sexy and sexual, as the books on the drugstore rack aim to assure me. I don't want to get around it. I want to live it. I don't want to "treat" it or "cure" it, though I do want to honor it with curiosity, and with "therapy" (*therapaeia*), attention of the kind one devotes to sacred mysteries. I want to allow menopause to be a

soul event, which means letting it be transformative, which means letting it hurt, which means really letting go of some still cherished old ways, accepting that some things are really over—though I may wish they weren't and may know I did not live them as fully, honestly, or courageously as I wish I had.

To learn ever more deeply that body-event is soul-event, that the two belong together, lies for me at the very heart of what this transition signifies. Most of what I have read about menopause disappoints precisely because it does not recognize that, speaks only of body or only of soul. I want to speak of the soul of the body, its within-ness, to go into the bodily events, the changes, the "symptoms," and discover their inherent symbolic meaning. I am persuaded that the soul meaning is not added on, not found through some movement of transcendence but within the physical experience itself.

The Greek recognition of the distinction between spirit, *pneuma,* and soul, *psyche,* is relevant here. Spirit seeks to free itself from the body; its direction is upward, transcending. Distance, clarity, abstraction, purification are *spiritual* values. Whereas soul is that which gives life, human life, to the body; it is the embodied self. The soul is the double, the *eidolon,* the image of the body that persists after death. Souls live in Hades, the afterworld, and in the underworld they are still recognizable in their bodily form but impalpable to touch, like smoke or shadow. That souls live in Hades says something about their attunement to the dark underside of experience, to loss, abandonment, failure, to unrequited longing and unfulfilled wish. To see with soul is to see the sacred meaning *in* events, to see them imaginally. The most essential character of soul is imagination — images are body become thought, thought become body. The soul is like those images of ourselves which appear in our dreams or in the dreams others have of us.

Although I tend to be suspicious of claims that we women have an easier access to soul than do men, I do believe that there are physiological experiences peculiar to women which may help us to appreciate more easily the interrelation of body and soul. Many feminists rage against this notion, and I share their anger at the crippling and distortion of women's lives sanctioned by the dictum, "Anatomy is destiny." Simone de Beauvoir, for example, sees the conventional identification of woman with body as the very source of her alterity, her alienation from self, her sense of herself as object not subject. De Beauvoir understands this identification as tempting women to passivity and to avoidance of responsibility for their own lives. Paradoxically, de Beauvoir's very passion confirms Freud's suspicion that the longing not to have a woman's body is a powerful undercurrent in the female psyche. That having a female body can be experienced as a curse is the implicit message of the euphemism for menstruation so familiar when I was young; "the curse."

Yet it is also a blessing and a mystery. This female body *is* my body. Living all its possibilities is living all my possibilities; accepting its limitations is accepting my limitations. To reject *this* body may be to wish to be able to repudiate embodiment as such and with it finitude, delimitation, change, death. That "menstruation and menopause are the physiological processes in which mild to severe discomfort is a moral accompaniment to healthy functioning"[1] may even be a boon, for it may make it easier for us women to recognize the inadequacy of seeing all discomfort or pain as antithetical to health, all pathology in negative terms. I remember how affected I was by the passage in Esther Harding's *Woman's Mysteries* which describes how the menstrual isolation imposed in many primitive cultures made possible the periods of reflective, introverted solitude, of withdrawal from extroverted busyness, which the soul requires. Menopause, too, may have its unexpected gifts.

I know that my recognition of significant transitions in my inner life is furthered by the decisive quality of the physiological changes which women undergo. As de Beauvoir puts it:

> The individual life history of woman—because she is still bound up in her female functions—depends in much greater degree than that of the men upon her physiological destiny; and the curve of that destiny is much more uneven, more discontinuous, than the masculine curve. Each period in the life of woman is uniform and monotonous; but the transitions from one stage to another are dangerously abrupt; they are manifested in crises—puberty, sexual initiation, the menopause—which are much more decisive than in the male.[2]

I experience the connection between the inner and the physiological as a blessing. Men live through analogous transitions but less dramatically, less connected to undeniable and precipitous physiological changes. Therefore, *feeling* the change, knowing oneself to be ineluctably other now than before, transformed, does not, I would guess, come as easily to men. (This may be why there seem always to be cultural rituals of adolescent initiation for boys which emphatically mark the passage—whereas the first menses may itself be regarded as sufficient initiation for a girl. It may also be why the so-called male menopause is often more diffuse and more confusing than female menopause because it is less anchored in anything tangible.)

To have the outward bodily signs must make a difference to the experience. To know so definitely—yesterday I was a child, today I am a woman; last year I could still have borne a child, now I know for a certainty I cannot—provides an emphatic reminder of the periodicity of our lifespan, a periodicity of which we are also reminded monthly throughout the years of menstrual flow. The radical discontinuities may also imply a somewhat different understanding of self, one more attuned to the appropriateness of being different at different stages along the way than the conventional equation of maturity with stable identity allows.

That old Abyssinian woman was right. A woman's life *is* quite different from a man's:

> A man is the same from the time of his circumcision to the time of his withering. He is the same before he has sought out a woman for the first time, and afterwards. But the day when a woman enjoys her first love cuts her in two. She becomes another woman on that day. The man spends a night by a woman and goes away. His life and body are always the same. The woman conceives. As a mother she is another person than the woman without child. She carries the fruit of the night for nine months in her body. Something grows. Something grows into her life that never again departs from it. She is a mother. She is and remains a mother even though her child die, though all her children die. For at one time she carried the child under her heart. And it does not go out of her heart ever again. Not even when it is dead. All this the man does not know; he knows nothing.[3]

There is change and repetition, not the more linear, unidirectional progression of the hero. Men discover this, too — as women forget or deny it — but I don't believe we women can as easily or as entirely not know it.

Reflection on menopause seems to lead naturally into general reflections on the stages of a woman's life. Part of the task of this transition I would hazard is such looking back, acknowledging what is being left behind, discovering what is being newly given. Helene Deutsch seems to regard the introspective, retrospective musing which menopause encourages as one of its typical "pathological symptoms," as narcissism. As I read Deutsch I am impressed by the degree to which she sees the postmenopausal years of a woman's life as essentially epiphenomena. To be menopausal is to be deficient, diseased, fundamentally superfluous.[4] (No wonder she discovers primarily "pathological" responses to what she calls "the climacterium.") De Beauvoir's words about the postmenopausal woman who has allowed herself to be defined by patriarchal culture are even more stinging: "With no future, she still has about one half of her adult life to live."[5] Though unlike Deutsch, de Beauvoir regards this as a *false* self-understanding.

Contemplating menopause inevitably involves us with all three of the seasons of a woman's life: the period from birth to menarche, from menarche to menopause, and menopause to death. It becomes necessary to consider the relation between this transition and the earlier one that takes place at puberty. Deutsch understands the relationship as essentially reversal, what was given in puberty is now taken away:

> The changes that take place in the body of a climacterial woman have the character not only of the cessation of physiologic production but also of general dissolution. Woman's biologic fate manifests itself in the disappearance of her individual feminine qualities at the same time that her service to the species ceases. As we have said, everything she acquired during puberty is now lost piece by piece; with the lapse of the reproductive service, her beauty vanishes, and usually the warm, vital flow of feminine emotional life as well.[6]

Clearly, Deutsch's view is determined by her equation of femininity with motherhood, her reduction of the menarche to the beginning of reproductive functioning and of the menopause to its cessation. Understanding menopause in a less disastrous way would therefore seem to demand also a more multidimensional appreciation of menstruation. Menarche, too, in our culture is played down, ignored, defined in terms of pollution and loss (but given indirect value because of its relation to fertility). Menarche like menopause is a passage that occupies us for several years; it cannot be reduced to one moment, to the first period. It includes all the years of anticipation and the period during which regularity of flow and ovulation are established. In the pubertal passage we are initiated into the cyclic rhythms of biological and emotional experience and into full receptivity to sexual passion, not only into reproductive capacity.[7] We are inducted into bonds of sisterhood with all women who participate in these rhythms, not only into the readiness for sexual intercourse with males.

Just as menarche means more than the beginning of menstrual flow, so menopause means more than its ending. It marks endings and beginnings, continuities and transformations. It isn't all loss, menopause is not simply a "deficiency disease"; neither is it all celebration, gain, and release as de Beauvoir implies:

> Woman is now delivered from the servitude imposed by her female nature, but she is not to be likened to a eunuch, for her vitality is unimpaired. And what is more, she is no longer the prey of overwhelming forces; she is herself, she and her body are one.[8]

Nor do I believe it frightening only to men (and to female misogynists) as Mary Daly claims:

> The menstruating woman is called filthy, sick, unbalanced, ritually impure. . . . It is consistent with the logic of the woman loathers, doublethink that the cessation of men-

struation is also horrifying. . . . When women become free
of the possibility of impregnation, one of the time-honored
means of imprisoning females is removed. . . . The postmenopausal woman is a potential escapee, deviant, crone.
Therefore she must be cured.[9]

To understand menopause as a soul-event means attending to
it imaginally, regarding its symptoms as symbols, and not being
surprised at its close association with underworld experience.
Deutsch's tendency to see menopause in terms of pathology has
a deeper significance than she herself may realize. She analyzes a
long list of "psychological symptoms": regressive longings still to
be able to bear a child, depersonalizing experiences of split
identity in which one feels simultaneously young and old, fantasies of shedding one's female identity and becoming a male,
the reappearance of long-buried homoerotic or incestuous desire,
lewd and shameless sexual exhibitionism, immersion in a fantasy world, being overcome by hypochondriacal fears. Clara
Thompson, too, though with much less emphasis, notes how
commonly menopause is associated with "lurking nightmares"
of "terrible somatic difficulties" and with "the spector of in-
sanity."[10]

I have come to believe that these strange longings and night-
marish fears are integral to the experience itself. I know I recognize each of them as a dream or fantasy of my own. My guess is
that this is not true only of me — that most of us (in large degree
quite independently of how we have outwardly ordered our lives
in the years since menarche) participate in almost all of these
"pathologies," even though they represent such contradictory
fantasies. Probably each of us alternates between "symptoms" of
denial and of exaggeration.

I also believe that the physical symptoms which often accompany the transition to irregular menstrual flow and its eventual

complete cessation (the hot flashes, headaches, dizziness, neuralgia) may have quite specific imaginal significance. As de Beauvoir says: "'The dangerous age' is marked by certain organic disturbances, but what lends them importance is their symbolic significance."[11] (The physiological correlates seem to be more universal than I might have guessed, less associated with particular cultural stresses and values. Still, it does seem that where there is clear social validation of a role on the other side of the transition, these discomforts are not experienced as symptoms, and there is less of the accompanying depression and/or excitation so familiar to us.[12]) To uncover this symbolic significance we may need to learn to view the somatic symptoms very much as we would view them if they had appeared in a dream.[13]

In my own case this demanded reconsideration of headaches by which just prior to my fiftieth birthday I was devastated night after night in a way that seemed to push me to the very limits of my endurance. My very matter-of-fact physician had given me a pamphlet about headaches which begins with a quotation from an ancient Mesopotamian manuscript:

> Headache roameth over the desert,
> blowing like the wind,
> Flashing like lightning, it is
> loosed above and below . . .
> It wasteth the flesh of him
> who hath no protecting goddess.[14]

As I tried to learn where the inexorable pain was coming from, a voice seemed to say, "Headaches come from the mother." I remembered my mother's headaches when I was a child, remembered how the joyous, brave young woman usually present would periodically be abducted while a pain-ridden, frightened, exhausted wraith took her place. In retrospect I wonder if my fath-

er's so evident valuing of rationality, dispassion, clearheaded-
ness often left much of her feeling unblessed. Her migraines
seem so obviously to have been connected with her menses, with
being female, with the one time each month when it was acceptable to be emotional, vulnerable, hurting . . . And perhaps my
headaches had something to do with the need for me, so proud
of never having been troubled with menstrual discomfort, now
to be forced to accept more fully that my femininity, too, en-
compasses vulnerability, fears, anger.

Yet although I see value in attending to the particular somatic
difficulties that may accompany our individual experiences of
menopause, I am still persuaded that the more important
"symptoms" are those provided by our dreams and fantasies,
nightmares and hallucinations. If we do not understand them as
integral to the full experiencing of menopause or do not discern
the symbol in the symptom, then the dreams are, indeed, likely
to appear to us as nightmares.

Because there is little in our culture to support such a symbolic understanding of menopausal dream and symptom, I found
myself looking once again to Greek mythology, hoping it might
provide some guidance. My search for menopausal rituals yielded
little; fortunately, however, there are myths which can help us
to an appreciation of the symbolic significance of the passage.
The major Olympian goddesses are associated primarily with
earlier life phases, with youth and fulfilled maturity, though as
was intimated by my dreamchild's receiving the name of Melissa, both Artemis and Demeter are relevant to the self-understanding of menopausal women. Artemis, through her sacraliz-
ing of all the physiological mysteries peculiar to feminine life —
menstruation, childbirth, menopause, death — and through her
modeling of a self-sufficient womanhood in no way dependent
on the exercise of reproductive capacity or on participation in

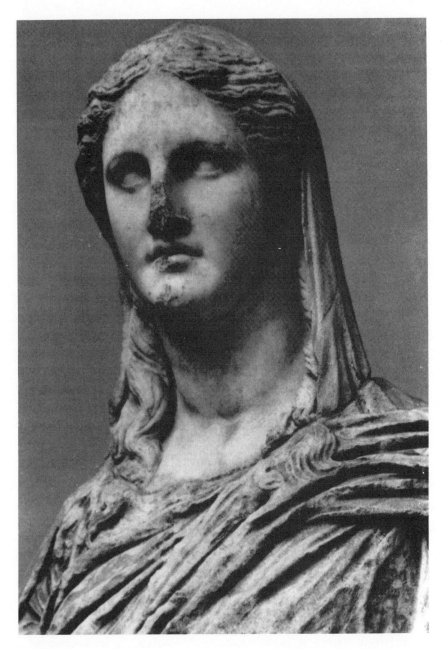

4. Head of Demeter, marble, 4th c. B.C.E., Attica, British Museum, London.

heterosexual relationships, represents the blessings which may be available to the postmenopausal woman. In her raging grief at the loss of her daughter, Persephone, and thus at the loss of her mother-function, Demeter displays a quite different aspect. Her reunion with her daughter and with her own capacity for fruitful activity comes at the cost of accepting the reality of underworld experience, for the separation will recur for a third of each year. (One thinks of Prospero's "Every third thought shall be my grave.") Yet there are minor goddesses that more clearly illuminate the polymorphous meaning of menopause: Hekate, Rhea, and Baubo. (We might note, however, that each of these three is involved in helping Demeter accept the loss of her motherhood: Baubo is the first to coax her at least momentarily out of her self-devouring grief, Rhea proposes the arrangement whereby Demeter might be reconnected with her daughter on a new basis, Hekate presides over the reunion.)

The association of menopause with fearful and despicable dreams is given powerful recognition in the traditions about Hekate. In Greek mythology nightmares come from Hekate who is herself a postmenopausal goddess. Hekate is closely associated with Persephone and Demeter; in the triad of Maiden/Mother/Crone she is the crone, the hag, the wise and dread old woman. Since an archaic definition of "hag" is nightmare, perhaps one could say: When we fear menopause, we are afraid of being hags. From Mary Daly, however, we learn the inappropriateness of such a negative evaluation of crones and hags. "A woman becomes a crone as a result of surviving early stages of the other-world journey and therefore having discovered depths of courage, strength and wisdom in her self," she tells us. Crones are the long-lasting ones. They are "haggard," intractable, willful, wanton, unchaste, reluctant to yield to wooing. Their strength and endurance are ugly, evil, and frightening to those who fear female-identified women.[15] The occasional confusions between Artemis and Hekate probably derive from their both representing self-sufficient womanhood, in-one-self-ness.[16]

In Hesiod's *Theogony,* Hekate is the goddess whom Zeus honors above all, who has a share of the earth, the sea, and the starry heaven. She is a great mother goddess associated with fair judgment and with victory in battle and game, with the fruitfulness of the sea, the flocks, and the human family. But elsewhere she is much more restrictedly defined as an underworld goddess. In the Homeric Hymn to Demeter it is Hekate who hears Persephone's cry as Hades pulls her down into the underworld and Hekate who lights the maiden's way back to earth and promises to see to it that the agreement whereby Persephone spends part of each year below and part above is kept. Thus three-faced Hekate is the goddess of the threshold between the underworld and earth, perhaps once identical with three-headed Cerberus, the dog who guards the entrance to Hades. She is preeminently the goddess of the threshold and the crossroad; her image stands at the entrance to every house and at intersections; the key is her emblem. Hermes, another chthonic divinity associated with entrances and highways, makes crossings seem deceptively simple; Hekate represents the seriousness and precariousness of all transitions. Like Circe (a Hekate byform) who directs Odysseus to the underworld but does not accompany him, Hekate watches at the gates. As guardian of the entrance to the inner world, we may also imagine her as watching over all that passes in and out of the woman's body: menstrual blood, seminal emissions, the newborn child.

In popular religion Hekate is the goddess of witchcraft and sorcery who roams the earth on moonless nights in the company of howling dogs and hungry ghosts. It is those ghosts we meet in our nightmares. Not all the dead appear as haunting spirits, only those who died too early, were murdered, or did not receive appropriate burial rites. Ghosts are souls who find no rest in death; sacrifices to Hekate are designed to appease the anger of the dead who were not ready to die. Hekate is present at those moments when souls connect with and leave bodies, at childbirth and at death. Her eerie following consists of those for whom this connection or separation was not properly accomplished; she is queen of those souls who are still fast bound to the upper world.[17] Thus menopausal nightmares may come from what is not ready to die yet, from that in our souls not yet prepared to leave the body of a premenopausal woman. (Another common "symptom" of menopause is insomnia. I wonder if it might reflect a fear of those same nightmares, a reluctance to cross the threshold into sleep, sensing its connection to the threshold into death.)

Until I started thinking about Hekate and her hounds, I'd forgotten a dream of my own about a dog whose howling went on and on, endlessly. At last I took up a sharp knife and cleanly severed the dog's head from its body and tossed the head near a garbage pail. But the dog's body was still alive, blindly searching for the head. There was no blood; the wound had immediately healed. I felt awed horror at the undiminished vitality of the animal. The dream represented something not ready to die, whose baying need had been driving me crazy. The body was in one place, the head in another, but the life (the soul) stayed in the body.

Harding speaks of the "importune ghosts" that come forward at the time of the menopausal transition, demanding a more fundamental confrontation with the dark side, our shadow, than was possible earlier.[18] This is a time for honoring our pathology, for acknowledging that in us which remains incomplete, fearful, and wounded. We need now, as Irene Claremont de Castillejo puts it, to "weep the tears which are still unshed."[19] The ghosts that follow Hekate ask only that they be openly mourned, ritually buried. Under her tutelage I see my dreams as providing me with the opportunity for understanding what my fantasies of pregnancy, metamorphosis, dismemberment, madness, disease, and death most deeply portend and what they promise.

My dream of being pregnant with the fatherless child who is destined to serve as priestess of Demeter and Artemis can be understood as an expression of one of Deutsch's pathological menopausal symptoms. She describes how often menopause stimulates "a strong urge to become pregnant and to re-experience motherhood." In some this is literalized, so that "often even against their conscious will, they give life to one or two lateborn children—before the closing of the gates, so to speak. One has the impression that even if sterility has already set in, it may yield to the woman's passionate wish still to be capable of reproduction."[20] Or the intense longing may be expressed in a hysterical pregnancy where the woman is fully persuaded she is carrying a child, or in dreams like mine which I carried with me into waking life.

The desperate yearning for a child is represented by several of the nightmare figures associated with Hekate, by Gello and Lamia who kidnap children and by Mormo who has lost her own child and so devours the children of others. Dreams of infanticide seem to express the same refusal to accept the loss of one's capacity to have a child. Thus Hecuba (in Greek, Hekabe), a recognized byform of Hekate, after losing her many children during the Trojan War, comes to reject her passive role as the grieving mother. She becomes a vengeful agent of horror who blinds Polymestor and murders his infant sons. Soon thereafter she is transformed into one of the fiery eyed dogs who follow Hekate. Medea, who invokes Hekate as her patron goddess, kills her own young sons when she feels herself rejected as woman, wife, and mother.

More often, however, the continued attachment to childbearing is expressed in myths or dreams about the miraculous impregnation of a long-sterile or clearly postmenopausal woman. The child born of such a conception is typically a divine child or one dedicated to a god, indicating that the birth is not an ordinary, literal birth. The most familiar such tale is probably that of the biblical Sarah, promised a child when it had long ceased "to be with her after the manner of women." The promise provokes laughter and smiles; Isaac's very name means a child on whom God smiles. According to the Yahwist's account (Genesis 18), Sarah responds to the promise with a laugh of bitter and incredulous skepticism which she then ashamedly denies. The priestly version (Genesis 17) attributes the laughter to Abraham whose smile connotes his recognition of how miraculous it would be for Sarah to bear a child at her age. The Elohist (Genesis 21) interprets the laughter as an expression of Sarah's deep joy when her son is born: "God has made laughter for me." Philo reads the biblical texts to mean that Issac was born as the result of a divine impregnation, and David Bakan goes to great lengths to connect the conception to an earlier passage in Genesis (Genesis 6:1–4) which speaks of the daughters of men bearing children to the sons of God.[21] Even if we see these interpretations as eisegesis, the texts clearly emphasize the contrast between Ishmael, the natural son, and Isaac, the son of the promise. Isaac's birth is a miracle, and his life is never to be taken for granted. The later demand for Isaac's sacrifice is but a simple reminder that he is a divine gift. The themes of infanticide and of miraculous birth are always closely related—the divine child must be sacrificed (though sometimes this may be represented simply through his being dedicated to divine service, as with Hannah's late-arriving son, Samuel). Even though Isaac's life is spared, he never really has a life of his own; his life is simply a less dramatic repetition of his father's. Isaac alone of the patriarchs never leaves Canaan;

he is forbidden to do so because he represents the promise that someday Abraham's descendents will be permanently settled there. Isaac is an intermediary figure, the sign of a future fulfillment. (In the Hebrew scriptures the call to sacrifice comes to Abraham, not Sarah, but von Rad refers to a Jewish tradition that when Sarah learned of Abraham's mission, she uttered seven cries and died.[22])

This ancient story explicitly admits that there is something ludicrous, laughter provoking, about the longing of a menopausal woman to bear a child and yet suggests that the yearning refers not to the realm of repetition and regression, the past, but to the genuinely new, the promised future. The transition from literal mothering may not be easy; it may be experienced as violently imposed. Before we are ready for a divine conception, we may first have to endure dreams in which our mothering (or our children) are murdered. Some anachronistic self-identification with our motherhood, some reluctance to accept the inevitable incompleteness of our mothering, our failures, our guilts, or our regret at never having had children, may haunt us in nightmare form. But the dream of a miraculous impregnation signifies precisely our release from the literal dimensions of child bearing, our birth into the new possibilities of postmenopausal feminine existence.

Even Deutsch admits that "after motherhood has ceased to serve the species, it goes on serving the individual experience." Old age, she says, adds a new phase of motherhood: grandmotherhood.[23] The difference between mothering and grandmothering is suggested by some of the Greek traditions about Rhea. What distinguishes Rhea from Gaia, the original creatrix in Greek mythology, and from Demeter, the goddess associated with the grain and with intensely personal motherly devotion, is that Rhea is the always sympathetic and majestic "mother of the gods." She is mother to the adult divinities who comprise the Olympian pantheon and thus grandmother to their children, especially Dionysos and Persephone. After the Titans have dismembered Zeus's son, Rhea gathers up the pieces, boils them in a magic stew; thus she re-members Dionysos. When Persephone is abducted by Hades, it is Rhea who comes up with the fertile compromise whereby Persephone may spend two-thirds of the year with her grief-struck mother and one-third in the underworld. It is also Rhea who persuades Demeter, still wholly immersed in her personal drama even after the reunion with Persephone, to make the fields productive again.

In the triad of Persephone, Demeter, and Rhea, Rhea is clearly the grandmother, purified of the possessiveness and the demands for heroic achievement which too often contaminate the love of mothers for their daughters or their sons.[24] But as is true of all goddesses, the many phases of her life coexist simultaneously. Rhea is not only grandmother; she is at the same time the young daughter of Gaia and Ouranos kept captive in her mother's body, and also the sister-spouse of Kronos, cunningly scheming to thwart her husband's attempt to contain his children within his own belly. She is maiden and mother, as well as grandmother.

Deutsch notes that "women who are good observers of themselves report that confronted with the climacterium, they experience a kind of depersonalization, a split in which they feel simultaneously young and old."[25] The mythological correlate suggests that this feeling should not too easily be dismissed as an illusion. Indeed, it may be when maiden and crone are *not* both present that the real danger occurs. It is Hekate's hearing Persephone's cry and later bringing her back to earth that assures Persephone's benign transition into womanhood and her reconciliation with motherhood (i.e., her reunion with Demeter, the mother). Hekate does not try to prevent the necessary Hades experience as Demeter would have. Just as important, it is precisely in relation to Persephone that Hekate appears as something other than a fearful, destructive demon. Maiden and crone need each other as surely as do *puer* and *senex*,[26] youth and old man, though the polarities are not identical. Where the senex represents rigidity, perfection, and order and is sorely in need of the narcissistic, inquisitive inspiration of the puer, Hekate the crone embodies a raging, roaming, unbound energy which finds its balance in maiden Persephone's self-enclosed passivity. Kronos as senex represents the unchanging; Hekate is associated with thresholds and crossroads, with transitions and transformations.

To literalize the sense of one's continued youthfulness may issue in ludicrous (though perhaps sometimes necessary) behavior, but to deny it is to rob our aging self of something it needs. Again that Abyssinian woman is right: "She must always be maiden and always be mother. Before every love she is a maiden, after every love she is a mother. In this you can see whether she is a good woman or not."[27] It is not only in goddesses that all the ages coexist. I remember vividly a dream of my own in which, after a long and exhausting swim, I pulled myself onto an island shore just before dawn and fell asleep. When I awoke, the day was well begun and I set about exploring this seemingly deserted place. I walked along the shore, marveling at the exuberant jungle growth which edged the beach and at the vivid tropical plants at the forest's perimeter, picking up and then discarding exquisitely beautiful shells of every hue and shape. At one point as I was walking I looked down at my own body and realized that my breasts were uptilted as they had been in my youth, that the stretch marks of child bearing were gone from my belly and that it was flat and firm. "Of course," I thought, "this is my true body and so is the other."

Deutsch remarks that there is a sense in which menopause is the reversal of menarche and understands this in terms only of loss—the womanhood gained at puberty is forfeited by the aging female. But in the traditions about Hera, this reversal is regarded as gain. Having left Zeus, Hera goes to bathe in the magical spring of Kanathos and there recovers her virginity. There is no suggestion in the myth that she recovers her youth or loses her memories of the years devoted to wifehood and motherhood, but in a significant psychological sense (and not only in the physiological sense that both are nonmenstrual) she is more like the maiden than like the wife, more her own person.

The *fear* that menopause may mean *losing* one's femininity which seems so strong in Deutsch becomes in de Beauvoir a *wish* to be released from the constraints of femininity at last. "It is sometimes said that women of a certain age constitute 'a third sex'; and, in truth, while they are not males, they are no longer females," she writes: "From the day a woman consents to growing old, her situation changes. Up to that time she was still a young woman, intent on struggling against a misfortune that was mysteriously disfiguring and deforming her; now she becomes a different being, unsexed but complete: an old woman."[28]

In many cultures postmenopausal women are recognized as no longer being only women, as in some sense now female *and* male, androgynous persons. In an essay on "The Older Woman as Androgyne," Barbara Myerhoff observes:

> In psychological and religious terms, the androgyne is equated with integration—human and cosmic. In social terms an androgynous role is a social opportunity provided to an individual to transcend his or her conventional sexually-stereotyped behavior, without labeling the person as aberrant or neuter. Androgynous roles are enlarged uses of human capacities unlimited (or more accurately, less limited than usual) by reference to one's sex. . . . While women are fertile they are of maximum interest to society and maximally restricted. The society has a heavy investment in their conduct; they must not only bear children

but bear them to the proper group, in the proper manner and time, and then rear them as proper men and women. When fertility is over, women may be left alone, and then their chances enlarge. New opportunities for individual expression appear, often for the first time.... In many primitive societies, old women are specialists in those critical moments when the designs of culture are threatened by a breakthrough of nature — birth, illness and death — moments when we are reminded of our animal origins and human limits. Women of advanced age are healers, midwives, dressers of corpses, and may be admitted to exclusively male realms which would be contaminated by associating with young women.[29]

Images from my own dream life confirm that human wholeness is often represented by some symbol of female-male union: the *hieros gamos* (sacred marriage), the male child within the female womb, or the hermaphrodite.[30] During that weekend devoted to intense preparation for my journey through menopause I dreamt of having come with my daughter to a small, isolated, somewhat dilapidated old house set at the edge of a wood. The yard in which we find ourselves is enclosed by high thickets and low branching trees and is unkempt; the grass has not been mown in years; wildflowers are everwhere underfoot; the roses and iris have long since rambled beyond the confines of the once well defined flower beds. The house belongs to an agedly crooked woman, a crone whose voice alternates between a gleeful croaking and an echoing warning. She appears a little mad; one would not dare to cross her. What she knows, she knows. I have come because it is time for my daughter's initiation, a ceremony which this old woman still knows how to perform in the old way. My mother had brought me here when I was twelve as my daughter is now. There are large wooden tubs here and there in the garden, set on stones which lift them high

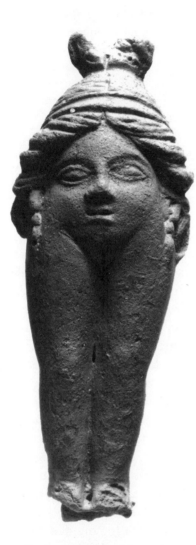

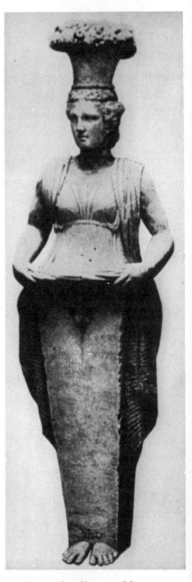

5. Baubo, terracotta, 5th c. B.C.E.,
Priene, Asia Minor,
Antikenmuseum, Staatliche
Museen Preussischer
Kulturbesitz, Berlin.

6. Hermaphrodite, marble,
Roman period,
Nationalmuseum, Stockholm.

enough above the earth so that a fire can be made underneath. My daughter and I set to gathering wood from the debris at the edges of the garden to build the fire. I think I remember the ingredients we will need to add to the water in the tubs (herbs, flowers, fruits), and I show my list to the old woman. She adds others which I'm sure weren't part of the ritual before; I question her but she is positive we need those other things as well. When I return with everything required, she sets about her preparations, while we start the fires below two of the tubs. Again I am puzzled. I don't remember that the rite had involved immersing first in one tub then another. But perhaps... When everything is ready the old woman and I gently lead my daughter to the first tub and carefully help her in. By now it is dark. She takes my hand and leads me to the other tub, wordlessly indicating that this one has been prepared for me. I am surprised, reluctant, but also recognize the inevitability of what is due to happen. As my daughter sits in her tub entering womanhood, I sit in mine not knowing into what I am to be initiated. The unknown elements which the old woman has added to the water have a strange effect. Their scent opens the mind, but they are also stimulating some strange growth in my body. I can feel the cells in my genital area growing, rearranging themselves; to the female organs which have given me such pleasure since I first really discovered them as I sat in a tub in this same dark garden years and years ago are now added a penis, testicles. . . .

I wake from the dream, puzzled: this is not my image, this image of the androgyne. For though I appreciate that menopause may be experienced as a release from the bonds of conventionally feminine behavior and from stereotypically female social roles, something in me protests interpreting this in terms of androgyny. That is to minimize more than I am ready to do the importance of bodies and of individual history.[31] I want to affirm that this more inclusive period is a new stage of *feminine* identity. I am who I now am precisely by virtue of having gone through the female life cycle. Part of the meaning of menopause as I understand it is the deeper appreciation of the soul dimension of bodily processes. Despite the physical changes, our attunement to cyclic rhythms, our enjoyment of female sexuality, our exercise of creative (though no longer procreative) capacity is undiminished. I am still wholly woman.

Consciously I reject the image of the hermaphrodite and find support for that rejection in the myth of Hermaphroditus. In that myth the female's longing for union with the male arises from her being a distressingly insufficient female. Salamcis, the nymph who falls in love with the young son of Hermes and Aphrodite, is "the only naiad unknown to the fleetfooted Artemis." It is said that "her only exercise was to bathe her lovely limbs in her own pool," comb out her hair with a boxwood comb and look into the water to see what hairstyle was becoming to her. Her assault on Hermaphroditus is desperate: she snatches kisses as he struggles to get away, strokes his unwilling breast, twines around him like a serpent, like ivy, like an octopus.[32] *Such* femininity may require complementation by the masculine, but I see the other nymphs, those who do join Artemis in the chase, as representing a more self-sufficient femininity, one closer to my own vision. Yet, evidently, despite the conscious rejection, in the unconscious I, too, image the transition to this new phase of feminine existence with this symbol.

A quite different symbol of the new life that menopause brings is the outrageously flamboyant female sexuality of Baubo. Deutsch names as among the "regressive elements" which often accompany "the progressive movement toward biologic withering" an "increase of sexual excitation" and "heightened sexual interest." She sketches a rather cruel portrait of the outwardly comical self-presentation of the woman involved in such a "second puberty": her ridiculously overpainted face and too youthful clothes, the clearly inferior admirers with whom she surrounds herself. Deutsch also observes that, just as in puberty, this resurgence of libido may be accompanied by a vigorous struggle against these sensations which leads to the sexual yearnings appearing as rape fantasies.[33] Such fantasies and nightmares were long ago recognized as included in Hekate's repertoire. Among her grim, uncanny attendants are the Incubae, orgiastic nightmares which stifle and outrage sleeping women, and the Empusae, filthy demons, so hungry for love that they devour their lovers. In Greek mythology there are also other nightmare figures, the twin brothers, Ephialtes and Otus, who seek to outrage Hera, the faithful wife, and Artemis, the self-contained virgin—as though women too long devoted to fidelity or chastity will inevitably at the approach of menopause suddenly long for a sexuality which they can only imagine as being forced on them. When femininity is closely identified with reproductive capacity, the end of that capacity may well trigger a fear that one is losing one's sexuality.

But the newly released sexuality may represent not the denial of that fear but rather the genuine discovery of a sexuality that transcends wifely obligation or motherly potential, that is truly one's own. The traditions about Baubo suggest that the Greeks were capable of greeting her self-indulgent, proud display of feminine sexuality with veneration rather than satire. When grief-stricken Demeter arrives at Eleusis, still in fruitless search of her daughter, she is entertained by the ancient dry nurse, Baubo. As Baubo swirls about in an obscene dance in which she ostentatiously displays her vulva, Demeter cannot restrain her laughter. Baubo *is* the vulva as she is also the wise old woman who is often given Hekate's place in the Eleusinian triad: Persephone/Demeter/Baubo. The myth suggests that the old woman can represent feminine sexuality in its essence more fully and more awesomely than can the reticent virgin or the reproductively oriented mother. It is too simple to dismiss the aging woman's heightened sexuality as only pathology or illusion. Baubo's spreading of her legs is regarded as a ritual act. She is often represented seated on a pig, legs outspread, holding a ladder upright in her hand; she connects us to the divine. The terra-cotta figurines which shape a vulva as though one could there find a face, indeed a whole body, suggest the radical autonomy of feminine sexuality — its fearfulness and its sacrality. (It is only fair to acknowledge that this obscenely sexual old woman is sometimes also represented as displaying not just pudenda but her most truly secret genital parts, her womb itself, and within it a male child. Thus here, too, the very epitome of female sexuality is represented by an image which implies that it contains a masculine element.) Baubo's vulgarity and Rhea's grandmotherly serenity may at first seem polar opposites, but the inner connection between these aspects of female maturity must have been apparent to those Greeks who identified Rhea with Kybele, the fearsome, sexually potent Oriental mother goddess, and worshiped her with orgiastic rituals.

The new, more insistent affirmation of one's female sexuality as self-validating, as complete in itself, as sacred, may also show itself in dreams or fantasies (or literal realizations) of homosexual passion in women who have hitherto consciously regarded themselves as entirely heterosexual. Deutsch speaks of how menopause may affect a woman's relation to her own sex. "Friendships previously loyal and harmless begin to be troubled; well-sublimated homosexuality is subjected to the same tests as sometimes in puberty: the sublimation is no longer sufficient." The woman may succumb to her long-repressed homosexuality or, even more frequently, to a homophobic panic which destroys long-treasured old friendships.[34] How much more gently Harding puts this when she speaks of the "autumn" of a woman's life as a time when a woman who has devoted herself to the life of a wife and mother can at last give attention to her relationships with women which have until now probably been left "in an exceedingly undifferentiated state."[35] The pull toward deeper relationships with women (or toward a more conscious realization of the importance such relationships have had all along) is, indeed, something many of us experience at this time in our lives, as we tend to yearn more for the intensification that same-sex friendships can bring than for the complement usually sought in relationships with men. The deep bonding possible among women is suggested by the joy that Persephone and Demeter give to and receive from each other when they are reunited and in which they so naturally include Hekate. Hekate's close association with Artemis suggests that the old woman's love participates in that respectful honoring of the other's in-one-self-ness that Artemis expects and gives, a loving purged of possessiveness.

All this suggests that after menopause the polymorphousness of our sexuality reappears; one may rediscover the continued presence of desires one has not lived. Deutsch refers to the reemergence of incestuous fantasies, now more likely directed toward one's children than as in childhood toward one's parents. I remember a dream of making passionate love to my daughter, kissing her lips, her breasts, her clitoris, and then being gently restrained by her from entering her with my tongue. I found the dream beautiful, not frightening. It spoke to me of my love for her and myself, my love for woman-ness, my joy in being part of the continuing cycle of love represented by women giving birth to daughters who will in turn have daughters. The dream acknowledges also that there are limits to our union.

The acceptance of limits, of separateness, of finitude, is clearly itself a central task of menopause. Something *is* over; someday we *will* die. Full coming to terms with our death is probably the task of the far side of this period into which menopause initiates us, not of its beginning. Nevertheless, from now on, "death and distance" are in the mix. Deutsch observes that the depressive overemphasis on the biological state of affairs may show itself in "pronounced hypochondriac ideas" which "in an overwhelming majority of cases relate to the genital organs. What was formerly a source of life now, in the hypochondriac fears, becomes a malignant growth .... Psychologically this expresses the devaluation of the vital organ, the destruction of its function."[36] And perhaps if we cannot honor the reality of the imaginal cancer, we might have to suffer a physical one (if we believe with Russell Lockhart that cancers are often an expression of something not allowed life earlier).[37]

A year before my imaginal pregnancy the results of a routine gynecological examination suggested I might have uterine cancer. During the week that intervened before we discovered I did not, I found it was strangely essential to live with the possibility, suspending belief and disbelief. It felt beautifully appropriate to be carrying my death within my womb, to imagine giving birth to my own death. Though apparently so opposite a symbol, its inner meaning seemed very much the same as that of my dream of being pregnant with my postmenopausal self. One of Thomas Mann's very last novels, *The Black Swan,* tenderly and ironically tells the story of a menopausal woman who falls in love with a much younger man. When her bleeding begins again she believes her youth has been restored; actually as we begin to guess long before she does, she is dying of ovarian cancer. Just before her death she tells her daughter:

> Anna, never say that Nature deceived me, that she is sardonic and cruel. Do not rail at her as I do not. I am loth to

go away—from you all, from life with its spring. But how should there be spring without death? Indeed, death is a great instrument of life, and if for me it borrowed the guise of resurrection, of the joy of life, that was not a lie but goodness and mercy.[38]

More frightening was a more recent dream of dismemberment. Fleeing some horrible past, I found my way to a fugitive band who lived deep in the woods among whom I hoped to find safety. Then I discovered that this group was conspiring to kill me and so I took flight again. But they caught up with me, killed me with their sharp knives, cut me up and made me part of a large bowl of fruit salad hidden in a refrigerator. When I (in some other aspect) tried to convince others of what had happened, they just said, "Looks like fruit salad to me," and would not look closely enough or taste to discover the parts of me concealed in the salad. It seemed hopeless. Then one of my sons appeared with a woman friend. They, especially she, seemed willing to listen to the whole story. I thought they would believe me, would check the salad, would find some way of re-membering the parts of me. My son, however, was soon bored and left. His friend, though, seemed to be really paying attention, until, suddenly she, too, got up and impatiently exclaimed, "None of this makes any sense; it's just crazy."

I awoke feeling that I really was going mad, falling apart, and that no one would understand, no one could help. I felt the compelling attraction of the imaginal realm as one from which I might not be able to return. I felt how radical is the break in my life that I am about to undergo, so radical that it breaks me into pieces.

But I also remembered the significance attached to the experience of dismemberment in shamanic tradition. The shaman heals herself (and in many cultures it is only after menopause that women may become shamans) by learning to tell the story of her initiatory experiences in a way that makes them relevant to others. She brings her dreams and images into the world of others. Helene Deutsch asserts that at menopause woman "ends her service to the species." I do not believe that. I believe that as we find ways of speaking of the difficult and deep and joy-bringing experiences associated with the birth of our postmeno-pausal selves, we do true service to our sisters and to our species.

III
THE PASSAGE

THE TROPE
OF TRAVEL

To the journeywoman pieces of myself.
Becoming.

—Audre Lorde

Initially when I undertook conscious preparation for the journey through menopause, I understood "journey" as a metaphor for a passage which would involve some radical physiological changes and whose full appropriation would require deep soul work. It had not occurred to me, despite my insistence on the correlations between soul experience and body experience, that the journey might take the form of literal travel.

Yet in his classical study of passage rituals, Van Gennep observes how necessary it is to primitives that their passage be not just symbolic or psychological but territorial, spatial; not only inward but also outward. To become a different person means (as colloquial usage so wisely admits) being in a different place.[1] The primitive in me evidently also needed such literalization. Albeit only half-consciously, I seemed to recognize the importance of a ritualized highlighting and bracketing of the transition. I wanted the focussing of a time deliberately set aside, of new spaces deliberately entered. To have continued my ordinary life without interruption might for me have meant some diffusion and evasion of the full experiencing of the menopausal passage.

I believe the essential structure of the experience, though less evidently visible, would be the same had I stayed at home. I believe also that my literalized journey brought me into touch with aspects of the menopausal transition relevant to others undertaking the passage in a less demarcated way. Just as our culture mostly forbids us the privilege of menstrual seclusion (unless we claim illness), so the kind of "time out" to celebrate menopause that my participation in a professional world which grants sabbaticals allowed me is but rarely available. Nevertheless, to attend closely to the details of our own experience in both its physical and spiritual aspects is a possibility available to all of us.

I seem to need to literalize and dramatize transitions more than do most people. I think, for example, of how important it had been for me at age thirty-seven (when my life fell apart after a painful love affair and I came close to killing myself) to leave my home and husband and university and spend six months in Europe doing nothing, except tentatively begin to live again. I needed the time-between. As seven years later, when I felt ready to leave behind the period of my life primarily devoted to spouse and children, I decided to move from the east coast to the west. Again, the inward transition required an outward expression. That I took a trip to the Orient to orient myself to the postmenopausal life phase seems in retrospect superbly apposite.

> Is it lack of imagination that makes us come
> to imagined places, not just stay at home?
> Or could Pascal have been not entirely right
> about just sitting quietly in one's room?[2]

I'm not sure there's *a* right answer to this question put by Elizabeth Bishop, but *I* evidently needed to do more than just stay quietly where I was.

Shortly before my fifty-first birthday I set out on a journey around the world with the hope (and fear) of being changed by it. Fully to experience the soul meaning of my passage through menopause seemed to require travel out of the ordinary world into symbolic and sacred space, open to the metaphorical dimensions of the places to be visited. Since the root meaning of metaphor is moving one thing to the place of another, it would seem obvious that metaphorical consciousness and travel are intimately linked. Metaphor reveals a dimension of meaning available only through a change of place. In terms of Paul Fussell's distinction between explorer, traveler, and tourist, my emphasis on symbolic associations made me a "traveler," one "moved by the exciting metaphoric relation between the current journey and someone else's journey in the past," by the relation between my own experience and the experiences of others as recorded in fiction and poetry, history and autobiography, painting and music. (The explorer by contrast seeks the hitherto undiscovered and undescribed, the tourist "moves toward the security of pure cliché.)[3]

The longing to relate the experience of my journey and my response to particular places visited to the accounts of other travelers was related to my desire to be open to the archetypal everywoman element. As I had written well before setting out, I wanted my initiation to be of service to my sisters and my species. I hoped to be able to contribute to the articulation of the typical features of menopausal passage. Traditionally in the rite of passage, though what one encounters is radically strange and novel, one also knows it is what members of one's tribe have always had to undergo at this particular life-transition.

I looked toward the new regions I would explore as analogous to the dreamlike landscape of "curiously fluid, ambiguous forms where initiates survive a succession of trials," encounter divine helpers, and attain transformative insight which Joseph Campbell describes as the scene of the paradigmatic hero's adventures.[4] I hoped to be able to respond to the sacred potentiality of the many places our journey would encompass with all of my being, attentive to the immediate circumstances of the present experience and to memory, fantasy, future purposes. I knew that our own preconceptions and questions, fears and hopes are fed by what we know of the prior response of others to the places we visit. These places already exist as part of an intersubjective world of culture, part of a universe of significance. But I knew (and regretted) that my sensitivity to such cultural resonance, allusion, and nuance was far less cultivated with respect to Asia than to Europe, especially Greece. The regions I was about to explore would be more radically unfamiliar than any I had ever been exposed to before.

Before setting out, I had recognized that traveling would require as reverent an opening of self to each place visited as I had given to the Greek goddesses whose honoring had occupied me so fully for the most recent few years. The etymological root of journey is *deiw*, to shine, the same root which gives us *deus* and *devi*, Zeus and Avesta. In his book on Zeus, Carl Kerenyi associates this root with the primary religious experience of epiphany, of feeling the presence of the divine as a suddenly appearing light, a full illumination *here*.[5] Because the Greeks were so acutely sensitive to the holiness of particular places and to the particular qualities of each holy place, they saw each sacred site as expressing or rather embodying the presence of a particular divinity. I, too, had come to understand how inevitably one would associate Poseidon with the steep cliffs of Sounion, Artemis with the Arcadian woods. I hoped that, in the much less familiar lands to which this journey would take me, I would still be sensitive to the specificity of spiritual presence potentially available on *this* mountain, in *this* cave, within *this* temple.

It has been said of D. H. Lawrence that his characters discover their identities through their response to place.[6] My hope was that my coming-to-birth self would be created in my engagement with the new places. I wished to honor them *and* myself, to focus on the encounter that would occur between us. I wanted to escape a narcissistic preoccupation with self, to be able to give due regard to the place where I might find myself, to its concrete particularities. Though I saw the journey as in a sense a trope, an externalization of an inner journey, I also knew that I wanted it to be a journey outside myself. It seemed very important that the journey be not only allegory, not only subjective. I hoped to discover my individual relation to the places we visited. I thought of how good travel photos are neither the ones that look like the postcards nor the ones where the travelers or their companions dominate the foreground but ones which reveal a particular seeing. In her collection "A Private Mythology" May Sarton includes poems inspired by her trip around the world, to Japan, India, China, taken when she (who like me was born in Europe and came to America as a child) was at the same point in her life as I was when I set out on mine. One poem captures particularly well the openness to the influence of place to which I aspired:

> The letters ask:
> You describe so much,
> But how do you feel?
> What is happening to you?
> *What I see is happening to me.*[7]

To be truly open to being changed by place, by seeing, I understood as a grace. How deeply Wallace Stegner understands this when he writes of traveling ("wearing a path in the earth's rind") as being "as intimate as an act of love."[8]

W. H. Auden once observed that for the literary imagination, "It is impossible to take a train or an airplane without having a fantasy of oneself as a Quest Hero setting off in search of an enchanted princess or the waters of Life."[9] But Auden is wrong; Quest is not the only trope of travel, although because the literary and masculine imagination have for so long been nearly identical it may often seem to be. The identification seems to ignore the difference between quest and pilgrimage, and the more pertinent difference between the courage to dare the radically unknown required of the hero and the submission to the universal rhythms of human biological and communal existence imposed upon the initiate in a rite of passage. The differences between the structure of the heroic quest and of ritual passage may seem slight, yet reflection on my journey has taught me to appreciate their importance. Getting past the kind of desire-driven questing that motivates the hero, that may appropriately motivate all of us until we reach midlife, turned out to be one of the most important lessons of my passage through menopause.

As Joseph Campbell notes, the archetypal pattern of the heroic path is simply " a *magnification* of the formula represented in the rites of passage: separation-initiation-return."[10] That magnification does, however, seem to fall more on separation and initiation than on return and thus to issue in a qualitatively different experience. Traditionally in the literature of quest and pilgrimage, the focus is on the faraway goal and on the dangers and difficulties of the approach. Arrival at the goal represents a climax and a turnaround point; the return voyage is almost anticlimactic, easy, swift, and quickly told. (I had some experience of that felt difference between approach and return on the only part of my journey which involved such retracing, the train ride between Bangkok and Singapore. In many ways the three-day train ride back through Malaysia and Southern Thailand was easier than the southern trip had been — I knew how to do it this time and what to expect. In some ways it also seemed less rewarding, precisely because less full of surprise or challenge.) Although the heroic quest is usually imaged as linear (or, as in Campbell's sketches of the night sea-journey, a semicircle), Van Gennep notes that among certain peoples ritual passage is conceived as circular.[11] I was intrigued to discover in a study of medieval pilgrimage narratives (which acknowledges that until the fifteenth century no Christian pilgrim had thought it worthwhile to write a detailed, rendered account of the return journey or to describe the scene of homecoming) an affirmation of the religious significance of global navigation: "Circumnavigating the round earth made one's starting point one's destination: The circuitous journey that returned home was thus combined with the one-way pilgrimage that symbolized human life."[12]

That my voyage was a circular one whose goal all along was home, became an intrinsic element of its meaning. Perhaps the affinity for the circular conception of life's journeys may be feminine, ouroboric, connected to that endless round wherein daughters become mothers of daughters; or perhaps it is simply a natural representation of the generically human longing for wholeness and completion: journey as mandala. Eliade suggests that the circular version of the initiatory pattern makes manifest that all such rites (with their affirmation that separations eventuate in returns, endings in new beginnings) seek to valorize death.[13]

It felt essential to travel in the same direction as the sun, toward the afternoon and evening of life. I had to head west, even after several friends had convinced me that practically speaking I would find the changes of weather easier if headed in the other direction. I knew I wanted to go toward the setting sun, to head first across the Pacific which I look upon every day from my study window. To head west was to complete a journey begun in childhood when my family had come from Germany to east coast America, and continued by my moving alone to the west coast in mid-adulthood. Coming back to Germany by way of Asia would bring me full circle. Moving forward from Germany back to my California home would repeat and thus reconfirm the earlier stages of my life journey. I had so often as an adult gone *to* Germany and then turned around to return; how very different this always westward voyage felt. Symbolically, I was recapitulating the earlier phases of my life but as part of a forward movement — a process I believe to be integral to the kind of retrospection menopause encourages.

That this trip around the world would function as my journey through menopause was not something I consciously knew when it began. Indeed, the full meaning of the journey was discovered through reflective interpretation — in this as in so much else the journey as a whole was like an extended dream. Despite my prior recognition of the mysterious interconnections between physiological and spiritual changes, I had so focussed on the soul meaning of the journey that at first I didn't even notice the change in body functioning. I had been away for three months before I realized that I'd had no periods since a farewell one in Seattle on the eve of departure. What provoked the recognition was the sense of my body being different as I was trekking through the mountains of northern Thailand — lithe and light, somehow more profoundly my own body than ever before, even in orgasm or childbirth. (When I got to Paris I saw myself nude in a full-length mirror for the first time in almost four months. I was very skinny, forty-seven kilos, and it was definitely a different kind of skinniness than when I had approached this weight before — attractive in its own way, but less muscular and less sexy. A different body which I began to realize would want and create different experiences.)

As a dream often echoes earlier dreams, so this trip was resonant with memories of earlier trips, particularly a journey back to my European birthplace undertaken thirty years earlier while pregnant with my first child. That trip had represented my initiation into motherhood, though I had not known when I began it that I was carrying a child. Now, in a strangely similar fashion

I found myself on a journey which would serve as initiation into a new life phase. It was time now to leave behind the life tasks I had taken on then. It was time now to undertake the passage for which I had been preparing with my dream of the mysteriously conceived child which I knew immediately represented my post-menopausal self. I had sought to make ready for her birth by addressing myself to those goddesses who might have the requisite midwifely skills: Hekate, Baubo, Rhea. I had not imagined that my navigation of this physiological and spiritual transition would take the form of a literal journey into a world where goddesses would seem unavailable. Nor had I imagined, after my invocation of blessing and support from other women engaged in the same redirection, that the passage would be one I would have to undertake essentially alone.

Because writing has always been for me so central a way of honoring and giving shape to experience, I had known from the beginning that I would want to write about the trip. Perhaps this is saying no more than is implicit in the relation between the two words, journey and journal. The conjunction implies that real traveling takes place a day at a time: it involves really being where one is and knowing one has come from somewhere else and is going on to a new elsewhere. Journey become conscious is journal. I wanted to be open to what each new place might demand, what each might reveal, and knew that the spiritual discipline of writing would further such multidimensional openness. "Places are odd," Paul Fussell writes, "and call for interpretation."[14] They invite our making stories of them.

The transposition of place into scene, event into story, journey into plot or ritual, inevitably involves some distortion, some transformation. The old adage, "He who comes from afar lies with impunity," reminds us that travelers' tales are fiction in its humblest and oldest form. In travel writing "landscape and incident do the work of symbol and myth."[15] Clearly the separate occurrences and settings of my journey would be given a particular meaning if set within the exploration of the trope of travel and interpreted as aspects of a ritual passage through menopause. Moments of the journey would come to function like images in a dream or episodes in a myth, which stimulate recognition of inner realities and changes.

Yet I discovered early on that the typically linear temporal form of travel narratives did not do justice to the felt shape of my journey. (This led me to wonder how many of the great travel writers have been women. Perhaps there is something essentially masculine about the genre as traditionally practiced, something that participates, even if ironically, in the heroic mythologem of Adventure/Quest, in the linearity of the Bildungsroman form?) The texture of the experience, its multidimensionality, seemed to require a different literary structure. The connections between events were more associational than temporal, more like those of dream or myth than like those of history. The time of the journey was a time that took me out of everyday profane temporality as radically as does a dream; I had almost no awareness of what was happening "in the world" while we were gone. Not until my arrival in Europe did I learn anything coherent about the Israeli invasion of Lebanon or the Argentinian defeat in the Falklands. Nor was there any better access to news of family members or friends. I discovered that these places, these encounters, these others resisted symbolic interpretation. Because I lacked the ready access to obvious mythological or literary association, I found the events of this journey meant deeply but they simply meant themselves—like the dreams we half reluctantly learn most truly mean themselves, not some lesson we might take from them.

The journey was one that took me out of secular time into sacred space.[16] I mean much more by that than simply that during the journey itself I found myself removed from the temporal pressures of my everyday life into a set-apart realm. I mean rather that even after my return I found myself to be oriented in the world differently from before: more defined by space than time, by being at home than by seeking, by recognizing the sacred in the immediately given rather than in some future discovery or some hidden symbolic significance. The journey taught me what I already knew (maybe menopause is a time for learning to *know* what one knows); that a woman's journey through life is not adequately described in the language of heroic quest. I think of Margaret Atwood's lines:

> This is a journey, not a war,
> There is no outcome.
> . . . .
> We're stuck here
> . . . .
> where we must walk slowly,
> where we may not get anywhere
> or anything, where we keep going,
> fighting our ways, our way
> not out but through.[17]

DEATH AND DISTANCE
IN THE MIX

*Always after the first thrills of
getting under way, the adventure
develops into a journey of darkness,
horror, disgust, and phantasmagoric
fears.*

—Joseph Campbell

I had sought to prepare myself for the journey through menopause in every way I could, but inevitably the passage took a form different from anything I had imagined. In primitive cultures, too, the potential initiate knows there is a passage soon to be undertaken and traditional rituals designed to effect it; he or she is attentive to all available hints of what might be involved in the rite—and is nevertheless surprised. The success of the ritual in forcefully weaning initiates from their outworn role depends in large measure on that surprise.

Having discovered Rhea, Baubo, and Hekate as goddesses who might midwife the birth of my postmenopausal self, I had planned to spend part of my fifty-first year in *their* world, in Greece, and in consonance with my vision of Artemis as a model of postmenopausal womanhood, I had planned to go alone.

What happened was different:

Tom looked mischievously across the top of his wine glass. "How wedded are you to going back to Greece and Germany next spring?"

I didn't reply; he knew I'd been planning the trip for several years.

"How about going to the Orient with me instead? I've always wanted to go and would like to go with you. I could take off from my practice for four months, or even longer . . . would you come?"

"Yes, I'd like to."

In the morning he asked, "Would you really give up your trip to Greece?"

And I answered, "Yes."

And so it began.

Or perhaps it began earlier. When Tom had come to stay for a few days after his father's death the summer before and stayed for weeks because it became so important to each of us to begin each day by sharing our dreams. Or perhaps before that: earlier that same summer when we drove across the country and discovered how easily we seemed to travel together.

It is hard to say when such things begin. We could probably trace it back to very early moments in the life of each of us. Certainly for me it was related to taking seriously the dream announcing that I was about to begin the journey through menopause. For him it was related to the task of working through the loss of his father. But the decision to undertake the trip together was made that wine-toasted evening; or perhaps a few days or weeks later (I've lost track), when we recognized that what we really wanted to do was not simply to travel to Asia but to go all the way around the world—together.

Together. That was central from the beginning. Alone, I would have gone to Greece, to Germany, as planned. Alone, he would have waited, gone at some later time. Not that either of us had ever gone much of anywhere with someone before. I thought I had, with my husband, my children, a lover, but those trips were more than I had realized always my trips, following my dreams, realizing my plans. He'd never traveled with anyone. At eighteen, at nineteen, at twenty-two he'd gone, alone and proudly so, to Europe, to South America, to Africa. We were a strange pair in many ways. He was twenty-seven when we set out, a year younger than my oldest son; I was fifty. I had been his teacher; he had been my therapist. We were not lovers though we knew that we loved each other deeply. We learned along the way that others needed to impose a familiar label on our relationship; to see us as mother and son, wife and husband, or sister and brother. We knew ourselves as friends for whom the difference in age and gender, in cultural background and psychological temperament, had at home been experienced as a vitalizing complementarity. By the time we left we had lived in the same house for almost six months and found it easy. We knew ahead of time that traveling together would not be as easy. We would have accepted the general truth of Peter Fleming's warnings about the difficulties of traveling with a companion:

> It is easy enough for one man to adapt himself to living under strange and constantly changing conditions. It is much harder for two. Leave A or B alone in a distant country, and each will evolve a congenial *modus vivendi*. Throw them together, and the comforts of companionship are as likely as not offset by the strain of reconciling their divergent methods. A likes to start early and halt for a siesta; B does not feel the heat and insists on sleeping late. A instinctively complies with regulations, B instinctively defies them. A finds it impossible to pass a temple, B finds it impossible to pass a bar. A is cautious, B is rash. A is indefatigable, B tires easily. A needs a lot of food, B very little. A snores, B smokes a pipe in bed. . . .
>
> Each would get on splendidly by himself. Alone together, they build up gradually between them a kind of unacknowledged rivalry. . . . Each, while submitting readily

> to the exotic customs of the country, endures with very bad
> grace the trifling idiosyncrasies of the other. The complex
> structure of their relationship . . . hulks larger and larger,
> obtruding itself between them and the country they are
> visiting, blotting it out. . . . Occasionally you find the
> ideal companion.[18]

Yet we innocently imagined that in one another we had indeed found such an ideal companion. For my part I knew full well that among those of my friends who were closer to my own age, none would have been prepared to join me in the kind of journey for which I felt ready. Few would have felt free to undertake so long a trip or one so little mapped out in advance and none of those few would have been willing to rely so consistently on third-class trains and local buses, to sleep so regularly in hostels or on the lumpy mattresses of cheap, fly-ridden hotels, to eat off market stalls or dare the local water.

Going together was integral to going at all—but being together was not always easy. In retrospect, it is amazing how very together we were, how (except for a few deliberately planned separate excursions) we spent most of every day and every night for four months in one another's company, only rarely sharing that company with any others who spoke our language. When I met my son in Germany on the homeward stretch of our trip, he had just returned from a month of traveling with his lover and wanted to exchange tales about some of the strains of traveling with a companion. "How did you do it?" he asked. "There were times I wasn't sure we could," I had to reply.

Even as we packed, Tom and I knew that in some measure we were preparing for different journeys. When we left he was still recovering from his father's recent death (what Freud calls the most important event in a man's life) and had just passed the licensing examination which qualified him as a full-fledged professional. He knew that when he returned it would be to reenter his world with the newly acquired status of a fully adult male, a role he both welcomed and resisted. Inevitably the trip kept reminding him of the earlier journeys on which he had embarked as a precocious adolescent consciously in search of self. Then he had seen each adventure as crucible, as test; then he had been responsible to no one but himself. He sensed that in some ways that image was now outgrown. He knew who he was in a way that he could not have at eighteen, and traveling with another would surely be different from traveling alone. Yet the image of journey as heroic quest seemed still the dominant one, as perhaps it often is for a man at any stage of life.

I came to recognize the inner meaning of the choice of this companion along the way. His masculinity helped me toward a fuller understanding of my own femaleness as something that could be known only in its own terms, not in the framework of heterosexual complementarity. His commitment to quest helped me to discover that I was no longer on quest, that I now understood the trope of travel differently. His identification with the hero forced me to wrestle with the heroic in myself. In a sense he was entering the life phase I was leaving, what Hindus designate as the householder stage, devoted to fulfilling one's social obligations in the realm of work and family. His standing at the entrance while I stood at the exit was just as important a dimension of difference as his being a man and my being a woman.

The details of my journey are in a sense beside the point, though no more so than the details of a dream which carries archetypal meaning. It is only as we begin to share with others—this is what happened to me and this is what I take it to mean—that we will come to know what is typical in our experiences of menopause and what is idiosyncratic. Only then can we begin to appreciate the polymorphous forms the passage may take.

Had I heeded more closely Esther Harding's warning that menopause may require a more fundamental coming to terms with one's shadow than is possible earlier, I might have been better prepared for how much my trip forced upon me a confrontation with my inner shadow and with my companion as projected shadow. When I first came to the retrospective understanding of the trip as a journey through menopause I wondered why I had chosen to live it in just this way—with another rather than alone, with a man rather than with women—why I had chosen to interrupt my work on a book on sisterhood for an unplanned trip around the world. I believe now that the interruption was necessary because there was something I still had to experience before I could be fully ready to write the sisters book, fully ready to let go of my premenopausal life.

I needed still to complete a reckoning with the masculine and heroic within, to finish with attachments and attitudes and unappeased longings that had been lifegiving during the period between menarche and menopause but which would be irrelevant and pehaps injurious with respect to the challenges of the last third of life.

When I said that I really wanted to live menopause, I knew that meant acknowledging everything in me which remains incomplete, fearful, wounded. As in my earlier confrontations with the goddesses, there could be no evasion of the dark and difficult aspects of the transition. On the literal journey around the world I learned how important it was to honor *its* darker moments, to respect as integral to the journey the times when I was overcome with fear, passivity, dependence, withdrawal, when I felt mistrust, dislike, or even disrespect for my companion.

My preparation had taught me to look upon Hekate as the goddess presiding over all transitions and most particularly over the entrance into the underworld. In the journey I actually undertook, "underworld" was transposed into "other world," but dread Hekate nevertheless stood at the gate, reminding me that "death and distance" were now irrevocably "in the mix."

Our departure was characterized by the anxiety, lonesomeness, and sense of dislocation typical of the preparatory phase. Tom and I had truly enjoyed getting ready for the trip together during the few months that intervened between our initial late evening conversation and our departure: reading travel books and glossy brochures, making decisions about our itinerary, getting tickets, passports and visas, buying one another backpacks that converted into respectable-looking luggage, deciding what to take along. But in the week or so immediately prior to starting out, each of us became very absorbed in our own outward and inner preparations. Making arrangements for my house and financial affairs, attending to last minute responsibilities to my patients, students, university colleagues, making time for the many tender and often difficult leave-takings from close friends occupied me more fully than I had expected. I knew I had lost contact with my fellow journeyer but was not concerned by that — after all we were going to have four very intense months together.

There were several stages to our departure. First, we drove to Seattle from where we were scheduled to fly to Japan. There I devoted myself to savoring the farewell ministrations of my daughter and several close women friends. I tried to pretend that, of course, my self-reliant young companion would easily take care of himself, but I knew that he resented my absorption in a female world which helped divert me from my anxiety and left him even more alone with his own fears. I saw and evaded his unspoken anger; I felt the man I had chosen to travel with had somehow disappeared — out of my reach, perhaps out of his own. The night before we left I had a frightening dream which seemed to continue endlessly, a Hekate-sent nightmare. In the dream we were lying together on a bed and then suddenly he began to attack me violently, fists pummeling my head and chest, fingers tight around my throat; I would half realize "this must be a dream" and struggle to awake. I would call out for help and find him there beside me in the bed, tenderly solicitous, and then realize in horror that the caresses were becoming assaults. I must still be asleep after all; I must wake up. I would struggle to call to him and find myself in his blessedly comforting arms and then realize . . . over and over and over again all night long. I still recall looking at Tom in the morning light, lying on the bed far across the room, knowing I dare not tell him the dream—and yet not knowing how we could possibly travel together for one day much less four months if I didn't. Sharing dreams, helping one another toward a deeper recognition of their more painful meanings, had been such an important dimension of our friendship over the years, but I could not imagine sharing this one with the stranger on the other side of the room.

On the plane later that day, I found I could after all. As we flew high above the Pacific Ocean, we were indeed in that neutral zone, wavering between two worlds, that marks the boundary between the profane world left behind and the sacred zone of the transformative initiatory realm. The way between home and Asia led in truth over "a threshold sprinkled with blood and water."[19] In retrospect, it is easy to understand that the rite of separation would require also a separation between us, a discovery of one another as strangers, a recognition that in its most essential aspects the journey was one each would have to undertake on their own.

But it was far from easy at the time.

It wasn't until I was on the plane that I really felt how afraid I was of what this trip might bring about, afraid of being changed in ways I was not ready for, afraid also sometimes of not returning, of dying—something communicated in some of the intensely experienced goodbyes that I had not until then been ready to let in. It seemed very hard, very sad, that Tom and I seemed to turn away from and against one another, as we had never done before just at a time when so much was painful and difficult and scary for each of us. The loss of "confluence" forced recognition of how at moments of testing each of us tended to reach for control and each experienced the other as controlling. For the first time we felt the age difference as barrier more than as creative medium. At the time it was terrible, very close to unbearable. We talked on the plane and that helped — we could at least still stand being together — but for days our contact was superficial. We were traveling together with apparent ease but keeping most of what was really being felt to ourselves. Both of us (though separately) thought seriously that if there weren't somehow a real change after a week or two, we might well decide we should each do the rest of the trip on our own. What really changed this was the pressure of preparing to do a dream workshop together toward the end of our second week in Japan. Knowing we couldn't work effectively together without really being together somehow made it possible for us, finally, to really talk during the hour or two before we were scheduled to begin. We both felt tremendous relief at the fuller reconnection made: when he listened to me give a lecture and beheld again the teacher he'd long ago come to love, when I watched him do therapy and saw him again as the truly gifted and compassionate, lovingly and stubbornly challenging therapist who had helped me so much.

Nevertheless there were many later times during the trip when we felt isolated from one another, unconnected, near strangers, though never again as intensely as at the moment of departure. To an extent that would have been unimaginable to us while we were planning the trip, we were each undertaking this journey alone, albeit so constantly in one another's company.

The essential aloneness may have made it inevitable that the actual other with whom we traveled was often experienced as a symbolic figure — as a projected form of an inner reality. My suspicion is that this is often true whenever we live through radical transitions. Our response to the others in our world transforms them into figures in our inner drama, and every interaction is experienced in exaggerated form, as though to highlight its symbolic significance. In turn, the other's sense that there is something askew in our response to them may lead them to respond in hyperbolic ways as they seek to force a recognition of their actual presence. Paradoxically, sadly, this only confirms our sense of their archetypal otherness. In the situation of our journey this process may just have been more visible than usual. I had imagined myself as having long since learned to withdraw projections, to disentangle the inner from the outer — and now had to learn it all over again.

There were moments when we deliberately chose separation, not out of anger or resentment but because one wanted to do something the other didn't. Tom thought seriously of staying on in China for a month of strenuous exploring after our relatively cushioned three-week stay. I knew that had no appeal to me and planned on going ahead to Bali for quiet solitude, for time devoted to dreams and writing. As it turned out, before we left China he had decided to go on to Indonesia with me. But there he did spend a good part of a week exploring the northern and eastern parts of Bali on his own. In India we finally hit our stride. Until then, there were still many days when his style seemed to me too active and domineering, when mine seemed overly sluggish and passive to him. When we learned to alternate days so that we would clearly know who was setting the pace and who following, these different rhythms became enjoyable — less dissimilar and less discordant.

By then I was grateful that we had risked taking the trip together and risked our relationship by undertaking it. I know it was sometimes at risk. I remember one of my sons once saying that he thought to "trip" together (with psychedelics) was even more risky, intimate, trusting, than to make love together. I believe that is true of the more literal tripping together Tom and I undertook as well. Many persons before we left had communicated their sense of how inevitably and deeply we would be transformed by journeying together. We had certainly ourselves felt the longing for and dread of such transformation, especially just at the outset of our trip. But as we approached its end we could affirm that the trip had both taken us out of ourselves and returned us to ourselves. We would be returning both as the same persons who had set out *and* as incontrovertibly other.

The early, painful moments of distance between us were intimately connected to death fantasies that are perhaps an inevitable dimension of as serious a passage as the one on which we'd embarked. As we left we were both consciously still coming to terms with our first intimate experience of death: his recent loss of his father confronted him with the challenge of taking his father's place, becoming a man; my sister-in-law's death had made my own a more real prospect than had ever been true before. We left, knowing that we would be completely unreachable during most of our trip should anything happen to his cancer-threatened mother, to my healthy but eighty-year-old parents. We both experienced the abyss that opened between us during the trip's initial phase as signifying the death of our relationship —and felt transfixed, unable to do anything about it.

As we acknowledged to one another on that flight over the Pacific, each of us at that point felt we might very likely die during the trip. We could joke about "death" being only a metaphor for serious transformation, but we knew our fear didn't feel symbolic at all. Certainly mine had been augmented by the many friends who had made a point of coming long distances to bid me farewell "just in case." (Indeed, two had given me amulets of protection. At a farewell party I was presented with an intricately decorated wooden egg that has been passed along from

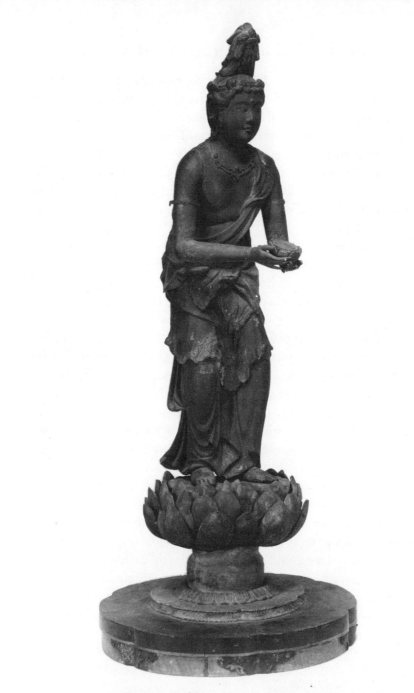

7. Kannon, Goddess of Mercy, Seattle Art Museum.
Eugene Fuller Memorial Collection, 36.23.2.

one seeker to another for over a hundred years and which, I was told, I must someday pass on in turn; the night before I left my dearest friend gave me his most valued treasure to wear until I returned as warrant of that return.) Tom and I found we needed to talk about the possibility of dying very concretely. "If I die," I said, "I'd like to be cremated and have my ashes sent home to be worked into the rosebed." "If I die," he replied, "I would like you to fly over the Himalayas and drop my ashes from the plane."

Our sense of death's impending presence was most dramatic then, at the moment of setting out, but in a more minor key it kept reappearing. Our host in Tokyo had a dream of meeting Death face-to-face in a railway dining car that he felt was somehow connected to my arrival. During one of our Gestalt workshops, I was deeply moved while working with an elderly Japanese man, both of whose parents had died of cancer. He himself had had cancer four years earlier and was terrified of its reoccurrence and painfully alone with that terror. Somehow he had seen in me another in whom he could confide. I didn't quite know what to make of these intuitions that in some way I was an intimate of death.

While we were in Japan our host sent us to Kamakura, to see the imposing seated Buddha, of course, but also to visit the temple complex dedicated to the Buddhist goddess Kwan Yin (whose Japanese name is Kannon). It was a day in early spring and the gardens were lovely, forsythia and plum trees just coming into flower and daffodils in bloom. As we walked from one terrace of the steeply sloping hillside to the next, we found that each presented us with a full-size statue of the beautiful goddess of compassionate mercy surrounded by hundreds of little foot-high clay statuettes, dressed in brightly colored aprons and scarves, some holding a doll or a little toy pinwheel, some with a toy car or train by their feet. These little statues, we learned, had been placed there by parents who had lost children—through miscarriage or abortion, stillbirth or crib death—and who hoped the goddess might bring peace to the infants' souls and to their own.

This temple moved me deeply; only later did I realize that my tears were not only for the young mothers and fathers visiting the shrine, but for myself. Only later did I see Kwan Yin as a goddess to whom menopausal women might also turn, to ask comfort for how in all our lives so much is miscarried or stillborn. I remembered then that further up the hillside there was another sanctuary dedicated to the same goddess, a series of caves which led us into the earth itself. Here, women came to light candles and to pray that they might again conceive a child . . . I thought, then, of my dreamchild, Melissa.

Although during the journey itself my dreams seemed to be of less importance than in other life-shaping periods, those I had were profoundly reassuring. I was not overly surprised that they were rarely set in the new, unfamiliar world which I was exploring during the day, but seemed rather to return me to the familiar world I had left behind, for I recalled Jung's remarking that this had been true for him on his travels to Asia and Africa. I also remembered how when I was four or five, recently come to America from Nazi Germany, I dreamed night after night of the people, the places, the everyday events of my life in Europe—as though to assure that they would not be forgotten. Similarly on this trip I often dreamt of places of haven and peace set in remote and little-inhabited parts of America.

One night in China I had a dream from which I woke with a sense of utter fulfillment. Tom and I were trekking through some steeply mountainous snow-covered slopes in the company of a group of Buddhists. At the end of the exhausting and exhilarating day we were ready to continue toward our predestined goal, but they urged us to join them in the retreat where they traditionally celebrated the completion of this arduous pilgrimage and we happily agreed to the detour. The place they took us to was high in the mountains, and though snow covered the ground, it was not cold; the air was the purest I have ever breathed. The building was shaped like a Japanese temple but open (or perhaps glass-enclosed on all sides), with tatami mats on the floor and enough white-sheeted futons on the floor for each of us. To be there was to be *in* peace, to *be*. I woke understanding better than I had before what it was in me that was *not* being nurtured in China and that I felt needed attending to. At the same time I understood, from inside, as I never really had before, something I have often taught — why China was so receptive to Buddhism when it was brought across the Himalayas. Our slow passage down the Li River and the lovely landscape near West Lake had both touched deep chords in me I would call Taoist — a sense of a *given* attunement to the rhythms and harmonies of nature. (Nature in the full sense of the "The Tao," not in the sentimental English sense.) Meetings with contemporary Chinese that opened into really *being* meetings had answered to a Confucianist-Buberian sense that being human depends on being neighbors. But something else which the dream suggested I might in shorthand call Buddhist, an achieved reconciliation with death and dissolution, had not been touched — except perhaps in the underground caves near Guilin.

The dream prepared me for Bali, where the ritual cremation ceremonies are such a central and essentially joyful part of village ritual life, and for India, where after observing the ritual fires of the cremation ghats from our Ganges vantage point, we saw a woman lying dead in the midst of the Varanasi market-stall confusion just a few paces away, completely unattended. In some unnameable way these experiences transformed death from a terrifying reality to an integral phase of ongoing life.

Meanwhile, we ourselves stayed well except for some sunburn, blistered feet, and mild diarrhea throughout the time in

Asia; but in Europe on the homeward stretch, as a kind of gentle reminder, we were both in physical pain — I with a pinched nerve that rendered my right arm almost useless, he with fever and a wracking cough that left him utterly exhausted.

The trip had been a kind of initiation into death. For him the first months after our return were marked by a deep depression as he was .forced to assimilate the lesson of the journey: that there are limits to what the heroic spirit can achieve, some obstacles which no amount of courage or energy can overcome, and that the hero goes on anyway, knowing this.

I returned a postmenopausal woman entering that phase of life which requires not just acceptance of our finitude but more literally of our mortality. The physiological aspects of menopause provided me with an inescapable reminder of the natural, inevitable transitions associated with aging and dying. Though there are moments of resentment and fear, painful moments, and a recognition that in all likelihood death is still many decades away, nonetheless, it (I want to say "she") has become a familiar presence. It's as though I'm beginning to know death as something that comes from within not as an external forced abduction, a death presided over by Persephone rather than by Hades or Thanatos. I think of Sophokles' description of Oedipus' death: "The underworld opened in love the unlit door of earth." I think of Rilke's Eurydice; walking with Hermes behind Orpheus:

> She was deep within herself, like a woman heavy
> with child, and did not see the man in front
> or the path ascending steeply into life.
> Deep within herself. Being dead
> filled her beyond fulfillment. Like a fruit
> suffused with its own mystery and sweetness,
> she was filled with her vast death, which was so new,
> she could not understand that it had happened.

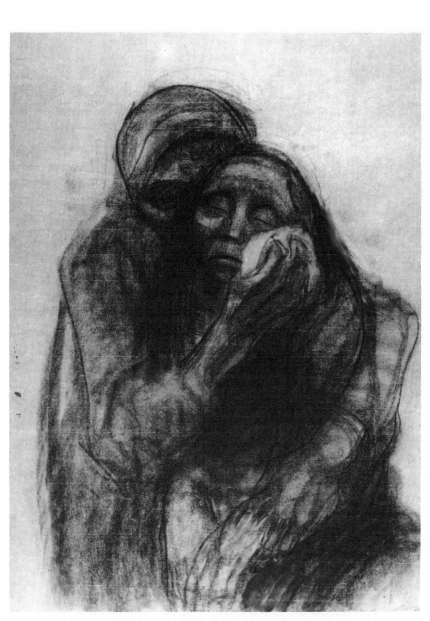

8. Käthe Kollwitz, "Death Comforts," drawing, Berner Kunstmuseum, Berne.

She had come into a new virginity
and was untouchable; her sex had closed
like a young flower at nightfall, and her hands
had grown so unused to marriage that the god's
infinitely gentle touch of guidance
hurt her, like an undesired kiss.

She was no longer that woman with blue eyes
who once had echoed through the poet's songs,
no longer the wide couch's scent and island,
and that man's property no longer.

She was already loosened like long hair,
poured out like fallen rain,
shared like a limitless supply.

She was already root.

And when, abruptly,
the god put out his hand to stop her, saying,
with sorrow in his voice: He has turned around—,
she could not understand, and softly answered
Who?[20]

I think of Käthe Kollwitz's powerful woodcut, *Death Comforts,*
in which Mother Death gently supports a dying woman in her
lap.

ATONEMENT WITH THE HEROIC

*Women you know Sir, . . . inherit an
Eaquel Share of curiosity with the
other Sex, yet but few are hardy eno'
to venture abroad, and explore the
amaizing variety of distant Lands. The
Natural tenderness and Delicacy of our
Constitutions, added to the many
Dangers we are subject too from your
Sex, renders it almost impossible for a
Single Lady to travel without injury to
her character. And those who have a
protecter in an Husband, have gener-
ally speaking obstacles sufficient to
prevent their Roving . . . . Had nature
formed me of the other Sex, I should
certainly have been a rover.*

—*Abigail Adams*

Before we left I had felt so clearly, "This is *the* person with whom I would want to undertake such a journey," but often along the way I misdoubted that feeling. Not because there was another whom I'd have chosen instead but because I came to wonder if there was *any* other who could really come along on such a journey. I who had spent so much of my life under Aphrodite's spell, in the world of with-ness, now had little energy for otherness, for relationship.

87

I had set out inspired by a fantasy of "Journeying Together." It had seemed apparent to me before we left that this trip would pull us into experiences of unknown elements of ourselves brought to life by the outer unknowns we would encounter—and also inevitably to unknown aspects of our relationship. I remembered vividly the impression Laurens Van Der Post's *Venture to the Interior* had made on me when I first read it more than twenty-five years ago. I had seen our journey as having that interior dimension he described so powerfully but also another dimension— dialogical, *zwischenmenschliche*, transjective—there is no fully satisfying word to name the interiority of the *between* rather than of the within. I had never done much reading in the genre of travel literature, but I was struck even before we left by how, among the examples of the genre I knew, almost all seemed to be the accounts of solitary travelers. I wondered if that were because only the lonely traveler has the particular kind of energy requisite for fully attending to what is happening without (and/or within) to issue in compelling writing. Or perhaps only solitary travelers need another with whom to share their experience so sorely that they in a sense create that other—the fictive, putative, future reader. Or perhaps it is because both quest and pilgrimage, the dominant tropes of travel, are essentially solitary adventures. For heroes others are simply helpers or obstacles; pilgrims may find themselves in company but with a group of similars not of structurally interdependent persons.[21] I knew of no travel writing that had taken the form of communicating what a trip and its various places and encounters had meant to several different participants—nor any that revealed how a relationship had been affected by undertaking a journey together.

So when I had first considered that this trip should be given some written expression, I had imagined Tom and me working in the genre in a new or rare way. It was a struggle for me to recognize how my imagined version of what we might create was itself a denial of "dialogicity," of my companion's real, particular otherness. What I had imagined was almost as though there would be two Chris's, a Chris-Chris and a male companion-Chris, each writing their accounts as fully, as literarily, as introspectively, as the other. Not pure fantasy, perhaps—there *are* others in my world with whom something like the kind of writing I'd imagined might be possible. But the actual person with whom I'd chosen to make this journey—a journey which after all I would not have chosen to undertake with any of them—was not among them.

We did write joint letters every few weeks that we duplicated and sent to our families and close friends. Almost always I would write the first and longer, more intimate, more inward account, and then Tom would write a kind of commentary or supplement. I had anticipated keeping a daily journal and then perhaps excerpting from it what might seem appropriate to share with others, and did so for the first week or less. But finding the right time, the right mood, the energy was not as easy as I had imagined. Perhaps when I have someone who is immediately present with whom to share impressions and feelings, dreams and questions, I am less likely to use writing to get hold of them. Certainly it seems not accidental that I *was* writing in the journal during the first days of our trip when Tom and I were not connected well and were each feeling very much alone—defensive, misunderstood, out of sync with one another (and, for me at least, with ourselves). Tom continued to write more regularly in a jealously guarded private journal than I—until he lost his book as we were leaving Bali. Perhaps that forced him from then on to share his more private responses with me instead. Certainly it was during the immediately subsequent phase of the trip that we really began to enjoy one another's company again and to recover some of our familiar intimacy and trust.

The letters were sometimes a subtle appeal for support from

those not present—a more muted form of plea such as those voiced in the letters to God in Alice Walker's *The Color Purple*. Yet it sometimes felt as though the primary "to" of our writing was the other with whom we were traveling but to whom we had not fully revealed the affect of the phase of the journey just completed. I remember how after an afternoon spent partly apart (toward the end of our time in India), Tom came back and spoke of having become aware of his homesickness and of a desire to write home. As he thought of who it was he most missed, he discovered it was me and the kind of sharing that came so easily at home and that we seemed sometimes to have forgotten how to achieve on the trip. I realized then how often the "to" of my letters had also been as much he as any of my friends farther away. Obviously, it is a commentary on the real significance of the journey for me that I would ultimately want to write about it by myself and with a focus on the journey as my journey through menopause. From the perspective of home, that is what matters most.

Yet that does not nullify the significance of his companionship during the trip. In many ways we were on different journeys and often each felt painfully alone, more alone than if we had actually been traveling separately. But I might never have come to terms with how much of my life I have lived in terms of the heroic model and how important it was to move beyond it had I not had to wrestle daily with a companion whom I often experienced as the hero incarnate.

As I noted above, I saw myself as a "traveler," prepared to delight in the metaphorical relation between my response to the unfamiliar and that of others who had preceded me, as I had done so often before. As it turned out, because on this journey such associations were not often available, I felt myself most often cast in the role of the unprepared initiate. Tom was self-consciously an "explorer" seeking the undiscovered, moving toward the risks of the formless and unknown. He reveled in the sense of being the first, the hero who undertakes a journey none has dared risk before. Often we could barely tolerate the other's way of journeying.

Certainly I often could also barely tolerate my own. I sometimes hated the me constellated in this particular traveling-with. Whatever capacity I have had at other times for with-ness often deserted me during this trip. Too often I felt myself going-along-with because it was easier. Too often I knew I'd probably have made a different choice if alone but could not find the energy to work at discovering/creating what the right choice for us (versus for Tom or me individually) might have been. In the vacuum created Tom made decisions and I acquiesced. Both of us got annoyed with my passivity. I felt manipulated and I suspect he did too—manipulated into taking more initiative, more responsibility, sometimes just more of the work of traveling than he really wanted. This surprised. Mutuality, reciprocity, balance had seemed so easy and spontaneous at home, and the little rubs and imbalances had seemed part of the human-ness of our interactions. But on the journey the full mutuality often seemed unavailable except through antagonistic struggle, and so for me just not worth it.

In the difficult moments of traveling we were different than we were at home, and the difference in one produced or exaggerated differences in the other. His inclination toward the heroic in times of stress aroused in me an unfamiliar passivity and dependence. We responded in ways that seemed all too stereotypically masculine and feminine as we rarely did at home. We became polarized; each saw in the other their own projected shadow.

I didn't like my passivity any more than he did, but I sometimes felt that what I most disliked in his behavior were aspects he valued; moments that left me highly uncomfortable were ones with which he was well satisfied. I was appalled at his delight in being able to intimidate the airline representative at the Tokyo airport when we had missed a flight and embarrassed by his hard bargaining with bemo drivers in Bali; I was dismayed by the stinginess he displayed in all financial resettling between us and experienced as paranoia the zeal with which he hid or locked his every possession. Yet to him these were simply evidences of courage, strength, prudence, of his ability to take care of himself or to get what he wanted. There were moments when I was furious and hurt at his unwillingness to recognize that I was older and weaker, couldn't carry as heavy a pack as long, couldn't as easily lift my bag to the racks above the train seat, couldn't climb as steadily at high altitudes. As, too, there were, of course, moments when I understood his assumption that I could do whatever was required as a beautifully non-chauvinist affirmation of my strength.

There were moments when I was grateful for his heroic approach, as when he was willing to take on our incompetent and patronizing tour guide in China and so win for both of us the freedom to explore on our own away from the group. There were also moments when I envied his greater readiness to take full advantage of such freedom. When I was "toured out" I wanted to be alone, whereas he could be nurtured by leaving the group and going after face-to-face, direct unmediated contacts with the Chinese. Like my mother he seemed to have a capacity much larger than mine for turning so openly, so interestedly, so vitally to others that they would share themselves with him as they might rarely do otherwise.

Often our interaction made me aware of how much of a hero/ rebel there is in me and how ambivalent I feel toward that aspect of myself. Ironically, my initial celebratory recognition of how easily I had moved through menopause had an indubitably heroic dimension. At many points along the way I had exulted in how well my body had served me through the rigors of the trip, and how readily I had accepted its frailties. During our trek north of Chang-Mai, I discovered with joy how easy it was to walk for hours on end with the backpack we took turns carrying. Yet I also found that climbing—especially with the pack—was very taxing, that I seemed to get short of breath much more quickly and intensely than I had anticipated. This made me realize that it would be foolish for me to plan on doing the serious trekking in Nepal that Tom and I had thought of doing together. Coming to terms with physical limitation felt like an important part of the trip, my first after-fifty adventure. It was on the trek that I first consciously realized that since we left I had moved through a significant life-changing passage. I had had no period since we left. I felt that in a very unremarkable way I had passed through menopause and was proud of how easily my body had managed this transition (as in earlier years I had prized my immunity to premenstrual tension, cramps, lower back pain).

It was not until my arrival in Paris that I was forced to acknowledge how much I fear and resent aging, especially the physical weakness and increased dependency that accompany it. Because Tom had stayed behind in Nepal, I arrived in Paris a week ahead of him. When I woke up on the plane an hour or two before landing at Charles de Gaulle, I found I had a miserable ache in my upper right arm. It hurt—a lot—and nevertheless seemed trivial. As it turned out that pain stayed with me for the rest of the trip (and for weeks afterward). It was caused by a pinched nerve which seemed sometimes to disable the arm completely and at night to invade my entire right back from neck to waist. The pain was, of course, often aggravated by my *having* to use that arm and particularly by my having to carry my pack. I asked myself whether I had at some point said, aloud or less explicitly, "I'd give my right arm for. . . ." It really did feel as though the

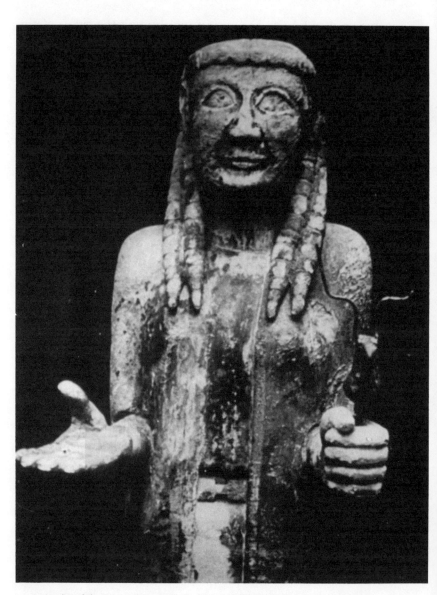

9. Artemis, alabaster, 7th c. B.C.E., Etruscan, British Museum, London.

arm itself in any usable sense had been taken away. In a strange way the physical incapacity was in large measure a soul experience, since it was at night when I was alone in bed unable to sleep that its presence, its voice, was most inescapable. The incapacitated arm was certainly a very pale version of the terrifying dismemberment dream I'd had during the preparatory period, but it seemed to have much the same significance.

The pain and the disablement made me aware of weakness, collapse, degeneration, vulnerability, limits, dependence. None of these were easy for me to accept as part of me. Although at one level I already knew that I was returning as a postmenopausal woman, I had initially experienced the transition in an unequivocably heroic mode. Triumph at having completed yet another passage, and so easily, had helped me to evade acknowledging the literal factualities of aging. While in Santa Fe in January just before we left as I watched my sister-in-law die, I had been made aware of the *work* of death (and the inescapable parallels to the labor of childbirth). Now I began to glimpse how much work is involved in aging—in allowing that process to be one in which soul and body co-participate.

I would never have learned how radically uncomfortable I had become with the heroic mode without the experience of traveling with someone so identified as Tom with the hero's way of being in the world. In retrospect it seems obvious that "my right arm" was both Tom and the inner hero I had managed to project onto him during the trip. In his absence I was having to confront the fact that completion of the menopausal journey entailed no longer having the hero to rely on.

I had invoked grandmotherly Rhea as one of my menopausal guides before I left. I remembered now how Rhea had depended on her hero-son, Zeus, to liberate her children (and thus herself, as mother). Becoming grandmother, leaving the maternal phase behind, meant transcending that dependence.

My anger at Tom as embodiment of a heroic aspect of myself that it was time to leave behind was clearly, at least in part, anger at its being time for me to leave the heroic period. The anger was a displacement of my grief at the ending of a phase of my life, an evasion of my conviction that the ending was premature, unwelcome, unfair (a conviction which coexisted with my readiness for the transition and my anticipation of the new phase I was due to enter). That nightmare hero represented one of those importunate unburied ghosts of Hekate's dread retinue.

The path of female initiates and of female heroes is different from that of our male counterparts—though the precise character of the difference seems still to be discovered. I am persuaded, though, that we do have a hero-figure in us and that menopause requires reconciliation with the heroic aspect of ourselves. I had lived much of my adult life in the heroic mode—questing, accomplishing, competing. For me (as the dream I had just before setting out implied) it was time to wrestle with that hero and free myself from bondage to that mode. For women who have lived the years before menopause in a more traditionally "feminine" mode, this might instead be the time to acknowledge and integrate their heroic capacities. Much in my experience seems to correlate with the "female rebirth journey" as this is described in Annis Pratt's *Archetypal Patterns in Women's Fiction*, where the point is not union with the opposite sex (as in the masculine quest journey) but a definitive separation from the masculine and a discovery of connections to other women as the source of transformative power.[22] That on the other side of our trip together Tom and I have had little intimate contact (though our friendship is again an easy one) suggests that the point of our relationship was precisely such a separation.

THE NEED
FOR WOMEN

How will we go on living
how will we touch, what will we know
what will we say to each other
                    —Adrienne Rich

F or many months my only experiences of intimate
connection with another were the often conflicted
interchanges with my male traveling companion. Our
interactions, as I have noted, seemed to lead to a
polarization of "masculine" and "feminine." I found myself
reacting in stereotypically "feminine" ways that felt very different from my usual modes of response.

Without such an intense dose of heterosexual interrelation-
ship, I might never have learned how much I need the confirma-
tion of other feminine presences to stay grounded in a way of
being that is receptive rather than aggressive or passive, that
remembers how and when to flow with rather than to struggle
against. Female puberty rituals separate daughters from their
mothers as mothers but initiate them into a world of fellow
women. My menopause ritual journey took me from my familiar
world of women; on my return I found myself relating to women
in a new, more consciously focussed way.

Though it puzzled many of my friends, in retrospect it is clear
that Tom and I, not being lovers, had more intrinsic appropri-

ateness than even we could have explained at the time: the discipline of celibacy is a familiar requirement of passage rites. It seemed particularly relevant to the menopausal passage — a kind of recovery of virginity (in that "in-one-self-ness" sense) without the illusion of youth or the denial of life-experience. The trip meant "time out" from overt sexual expression, as from so much else. It was a time "between" comparable to the time in Demeter's life between Persephone's disappearance and her reappearance on a different basis, the time when Demeter meets Baubo. Baubo flaunted her sexuality, mine became quiescent; yet I sense that the meaning of my holding my sexuality within and of Baubo's so boldly manifesting hers is much the same. I was reclaiming my sexuality as my own. On my return I would begin to let it out again but very differently from before.

Yet honesty requires acknowledgment that the lack of sexual interaction sometimes felt not like choice but imposition — and rejection. It was a new experience for me not to be desired by a man with whom I was on intimate terms and painful to admit that it was because I was too old. Wrinkles, flaccid skin, slightly thickened waist rendered me erotically invisible! How vividly this recalled the menopausal heroine of Doris Lessing's *Summer Before the Dark* who found herself invisible to the same men who would approvingly whistle at her when she got herself youthfully "dolled up." Leaving behind an image of self dependent on heterosexual affirmation inspired the same passionate ambivalence that I felt toward the other changes associated with menopause.

The lack of contact with women was even more painful. In some instances, my traveling with a male companion seemed to make me seem less approachable to women who might otherwise have confided in me. In China, I found that on the rare occasions when I wandered through the sidestreets by myself, young women would shyly stop me to ask if we could talk in

English for a while. Several times when Tom left me sitting alone during the train ride through Malaysia, I was pounced on by a group of young women who had clearly been waiting for just such an opportunity. With no man around they were willing to talk candidly and personally about their family interactions, their ambitions, their frustrations. In such situations I found that naming my interest in sister bonds almost always evoked lively and seriously reflective conversation. But more typical were my experiences on trains in India. Most of our fellow passengers would be traveling in family groups, usually consisting of a middle-class, fairly well-educated, English-speaking father, his typically much younger, shy, quiet wife and their *many* young children. Often an extended family would be going on holiday together: several middle-aged brothers with their wives and children. Most of my conversations would be with the men. The women almost never knew any English and (so the men would tell me) had had little education. "She is a good woman and good mother but I cannot talk to her." Women in Asia share even less of their inner lives with men than we do, live almost entirely in a female world; what the men said of them told me nothing of their experience of their lives. Perhaps if I had come to India when I was younger in the company of my own small children, I might have found some way of communicating with the women, of suggesting how much as women we did have in common. But though there were some shared smiles, especially over the children's doings, there was little sense of real contact. I came more and more to feel the lack of contact with women as something palpably missing—almost like an organ of my own that had been amputated. Years ago, I remembered, a male colleague had spoken of his regret while in India at being cut off from any contact with women. Because I had assumed that this deprivation was due to Indian taboos against contra-sexual emotional intimacy, it had never occurred to me I would suffer the same loss.

The one experience we had of a culture where the women dominated and were more friendly and available than the men was in the hill country of Northern Thailand. The first tribe we visited was, we were told, the only matrilocal, matrifocal one. Its men have the reputation of being doped up with opium most of the time; once a year they go to pick the opium grown by another tribe in sufficient quantity to earn enough to keep their own habit supplied. It seemed a sad story—who could say whether the women's dominance created the men's passivity or whether the women took charge because the men didn't.

When we visited the Grand Palace in Bangkok, we had an unexpected experience of the veneration paid feminine divinity in Asia. Just as we were about to leave the palace compound, we saw a large crowd gathered expectantly on two sides of a promenade. We joined them, and soon discovered the cause of the excitement: a goddess, a divine being even more powerful than Lord Buddha himself, the creatrix of the Thai land and people, was about to be carried in a processional. The ritual was one celebrated only once every fifty years and so for almost everyone present something never before witnessed. How amazing when her palladin appeared to discover that SHE was only seven or eight inches tall!

Of course in India we were often exposed to rituals and temples dedicated to goddesses, though I will never forget the endlessly long hike through the heat of mid-day Benares to its fabled Durga temple—and discovering when we at last arrived that its precincts were closed to women. There was painfully little on this trip to assuage my longing for the kind of intimate personal interchange with women which could support my attempt to stay in touch with my own feminine strengths. No wonder I was so moved by one of the few books I read while on the trip, E. M. Broner's *A Weave of Women*. The title describes the book wonderfully: it is a weaving of event, ritual, fantasy—Jewish, feminist — wonderfully fresh and new but full of the most ancient rhythms and motifs of storytelling. It was joyously comic, wisely tragic, in that sense full of genuine *Yiddishkeit*. I felt it had been written for me, felt my life interwoven with those of the powerful, generous women whose stories the book presents. I did something I have never done before: I began rereading immediately upon finishing the last chapter!

No wonder, either, that I was so taken with the woman in whose suburban Parisian house I stayed during my first week in Europe. Though she was a stranger (friend of a friend), I felt at home with her immediately and was flooded with gratitude at being with a *woman* again. The recognition brought me to the edge of tears often in the next few days. I loved her combination of maturity and vitality, the way her beauty seemed to come from the fullness of her forty years rather than as a denial of them. Though so generously available to me, she nevertheless communicated that she was essentially a woman of deep reserve. The few days I spent with her were, simply, a blessing.

My return home became in a singularly important way a return home to women. The months of separation from them served as an initiation into a life phase where I recognize the primacy of my relationship to women more clearly than ever before.

ALONG THE WAY

*Where we had thought to travel outward,
we shall come to the center of our own
existence. . . . The passage may be over-
ground, incidentally; fundamentally it
is inward — into depths where obscure
resistances are overcome and long lost,
forgotten powers revivified.*
— Joseph Campbell

O ur journey taught me to appreciate the intimate connection between travel and travail. For me the connection implied the labor implicit in all birthgiving; for
Tom the travail referred to the difficult and often
toilsome challenges, the anxiety and hard work, discomfort and
danger that confront the hero. His conception certainly took account of the fact that "travel" derives from a term describing a
medieval instrument of torture! It often seemed to me that for
him nothing was worth doing unless it was hard. (Even when
we had found a hotel room that was within our budget and
clean and quiet enough to be acceptable, he wouldn't agree to
take it no matter how tired or hungry we might be until we'd
made sure it was the very best deal in town.) Whereas it was
(and is) my sense that life brings enough tests on its own without our having to go looking for gratuitous ones. Often I wanted
to echo Atwood's Circe, "Don't you ever get tired of saying
onward?"

We had come in search of sacred experience and, of course,

learned that unless we are open to it, no place can reveal its sacredness. During our first week in Japan I *knew* the beauty of the alpine landscape and the Kyoto gardens we visited but couldn't *feel* it. Sarton writes of a similar response during her first weeks in Japan:

> Now it is coming to an end,
> I see how I have lived,
> Observing, recording
> With a painter's impersonal eye:
> Plum Blossom,
> White butterflies
> Against a dark pine.
> That feathery elegance, bamboo.
> That fabulous mountain, a small rock.
>
> So it has been for three weeks,
> Until a single tired face,
> The face of a servant,
> Broke the pane of glass
> Between me and all things:
> I am inside the landscape....
>
> The poems begin here.[23]

We had come in search of sacred experience and, of course, learned how inevitably it is intertwined with the profane, the ordinary, the distracting, the unpleasant. I can remember, for example, visiting the rock garden at Ryonji in Kyoto on a Sunday afternoon. It was mobbed with chattering tourists. (It helped only a little that they were Japanese rather than American.) We were accosted by the continual blare of a loudspeaker describing the beauty and peace symbolized by the placement of the rocks on the sand. We could sense that tranquillity—but only by an act of forceful bracketing and imagining that I still wish hadn't been necessary.

We hated Hong Kong which felt to us like one enormous shopping mall—or sometimes like Disneyland. In China, we were repelled by the tourism of the group we were traveling with whose primary interests seemed to be shopping and eating. Few of them seemed to have any interest in direct contact with individual Chinese, in checking out the tour guides' version of contemporary China, or having any experiences of China beyond the prepackaged ones arranged for us. Yet we found that the "real" China *was* available to us. I recall especially an early evening stroll in Guilin through the narrow little alleyways along which people live. Because it was Sunday, these alleys were full of people of all ages enjoying themselves and of others making a little extra money—selling produce or the cheap little odds and ends that show up at such makeshift sidewalk stalls anywhere in the world, washing clothes in company, or repairing bikes, mending clothes, making little things out of discards and scraps. We were the only westerners present and at least as fascinating to the Chinese as they to us.

Whenever we would pause a crowd would gather to see what had attracted us. We stood for a long while watching two men, squatting before two old wooden boxes, one hammering assiduously to flatten out a little strip of metal; the other, as patiently, cutting a design into an already flattened strip and shaping it into a ring. Actually, it took us quite a while to figure out just what they were making but we loved the quality of how they were doing it: their total absorption and yet pleased delight in being watched not only by us but by the much larger crowd that had gathered since our arrival. I found myself as attentive to the entire scene as to the two craftsmen, and shared broad grins and bubbly little "hel-lo's" with the children and shy smiles with the women. Every once in a while the elder of the two "jewelers" would look up at Tom, appreciating *his* appreciation, and before we left, quietly and simply, without any words at all he took an already fashioned ring from his own finger and gave it to Tom. The gesture touched, awed not only us but everyone present—an enormously generous giving that came from him but in a sense also from the whole assembled company—and, I felt, in some way, from *China*.

Paradigmatic of being underway were, of course, the many hours and days we spent in trains and buses. (We once figured that over half of our time in India was spent in transit from one place to another!) Typically, we enjoyed traveling third-class and usually being the only westerners to do so. I loved the contrast between having slept in the very posh Hotel Furama in Hong Kong one night (courtesy of our China tour) and finding myself spending the next lying on some newspapers spread out under the third-class seats of the train making its way through Southern Thailand. Yet there were times, especially in India, when this mode of travel was almost too much, even for us. Having failed to get reservations for the fifteen-hour trip to Kashmir, we decided to take the train nonetheless, since the chances of getting reservations for the next day's train seemed little better—and so began what became *the* train adventure of our entire trip. The unreserved car was so packed that there was no way of even opening the door to try to squeeze some room for ourselves. For a time, those in one of the reserved cars happily made space for us until an officious conductor chased us away. (We'd been assured, wrongly as it turned out, that a little "baksheech" would take care of such an eventuality.) We went from car to car, trying to make ourselves as inconspicuous as possible, but the conductors seemed determined not to permit any irregularity; each sent us to some other part of the train from which we would in turn be chased. As the train finally began to take off from the station where it had come to seem eternally moored, we were on the platform. We each desperately pushed ourselves through the nearest door. I found myself in an all-military car whose occupants had at first tried to keep me out but then were so amused by my determination that they hid me all night. Tom was in a first-class coach and ended up spending most of the night hiding from the conductor in a lavatory! Somehow in the confusion we had ended up with one another's backpacks; I had all the money and both our passports; he had the train tickets. Neither of us knew what had happened to the other, and we somehow missed each other when we got off the train in Jammu mid-afternoon the next day. What a nightmare of separation, of finding that there is no place anywhere where you rightfully belong. You can easily imagine the relief—and delight—of our reconnection.

Though we agreed we'd not travel again on an Indian train for so long a trip without reservations, our commitment to not traveling tourist-style remained firm. We were in search of adventure and metaphor, of the sacred and the transformative. The impatience with tourism expressed our desire to get away from the profane, to expose ourselves to places whose holiness was fundamental to cultures other than our own and to seemingly ordinary places whose numinous power might be self-validating to us.

Often on our trip we found ourselves in landscapes eerily familiar and deeply moving, landscapes that were like paintings or like dreams become actual. This was especially true in southwest China. We spent one day on a boat following the Li River as it makes its way past the mountains peculiar to this area, the irregularly rounded-off pyramidal mountains jutting up from the flat valleys made familiar in so much Chinese landscape painting. We were taken on a slow passage through a gently beautiful terrain—a transportation into those paintings and into their peace. Some scenes touched primordial memories. In that same part of China, near Guilin, we were taken to the hillside caves on the outskirts of the city, a seemingly endless under-world labyrinth. The high narrow passageways opened into chamber after chamber filled with fantastically shaped stalactites and stalagmites. We were easily able to separate ourselves from guide and group and make our way through this wonderland together —a truly otherworldly realm—as foreign yet familiar as when one first snorkels or scuba-dives and enters the undersea world. I felt myself both in some archaic, ancient, always-there space, deep inside inside-ness, and also in some futuristic realm existing only in fantasy. The sense of going in, deeper and deeper, endlessly, had the intense reality of dream experience. Then, with no preparation, we suddenly found ourselves at the edge of a vast underground dome-shaped chamber, a space larger than any cathedral whose sacredness was palpable. Different from any space I had ever been in, not only in appearance but in effect, the closest I had ever come before to the particular quality of this experience had been while sitting alone in a large kiva at Chaco Canyon. One could easily imagine the people who lived near these caves gathering here both in hushed and ecstatic ritual. Whether this ever literally happened at this place seemed irrelevant to my knowledge that it *had*.

It was in India more than anywhere else that we were forced to deal with the *work* of travel, to walk what Campbell calls "the road of trials"—an opus I have come to see as preparatory to submitting myself to the *work* of aging, the work of dying. The basic experience was of always being caught off guard, of being tripped, mauled, and then caressed. Having arrived in Delhi late in the afternoon, we made our way into town by public bus and found a relatively cheap hotel on a bustling road full of food and clothing stalls called, not too surprisingly, Market Road. Tom was exhausted and went right to sleep but I walked around the immediate neighborhood for a few hours before dusk, getting a preliminary taste of India. I loved Delhi that first night. It was all so much as I had imagined it—the vitality of the bustling crowds, the cows unconcernedly meandering through the streets, the people preparing to sleep on the sidewalks, the gossamer saris lending grace to the most tawdry scene, the utter peace and silence in the gardens of the Ramakrishna mission just a half block away, the tantalizing spicy smells. All of this seemed so emphatically, indubitably India. I felt embraced and ready to embrace, and that first evening imagined I could do so at my own pace. The next morning I began to discover the illusoriness of this conviction. For India accosts and withdraws. *She*, not we, determines the rhythm. The destructive and the creative, malign and benign energies seemed inextricably and inexplicably intertwined.

I think India might have taught me the primacy of Kali's divinity quite apart from my ever having known this goddess's name. Over and over again, just as we found ourselves basking in our delight in being in India she knocked us flat. Then when we were full of exhaustion, frustration, anger, something so unexpectedly lovely and soul-satisfying would happen that everything else was wiped away. To say only "I love India" or only "I hate her" was inconceivable; either statement alone would have seemed a grossly dishonest sentimentality.

Though my preparation for menopause had focussed on attending to what illumination of the experience such Greek goddesses as Rhea, Baubo, and Hekate might provide, these goddesses (not too surprisingly) often seemed irrelevant during my time in the Orient. Leaving my familiar world seemed to entail leaving behind those divinities upon whose guidance I had come to depend. The highly differentiated goddesses of the Greek pantheon had helped me sort through the different aspects of my own female being. Evidently it was now time to confront again the more fearful power of the undifferentiated feminine. One

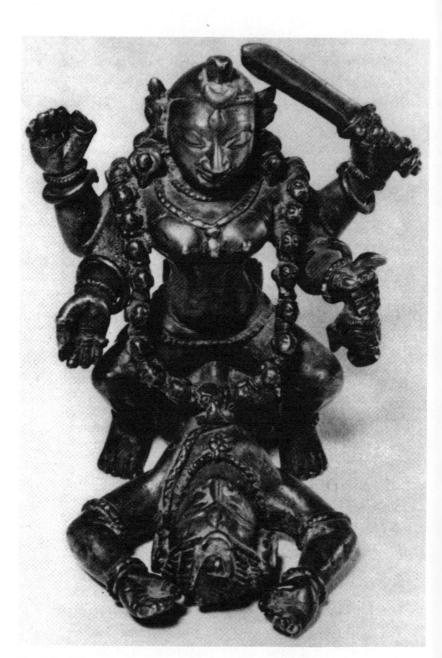

10. Kali, 17th c. bronze, Orissa, New York Graphic Society.

of Her embodiments is Kali, a goddess who forces upon us recognition of the absurd fragility of all social order and of the terrifying inescapability of death. Kali is more filled with primary generative energy than Rhea, more ravenous in her sexual appetite than Baubo, far darker than Hekate. To turn to her is to confront untamed female power, to realize that now when one's focus is no longer on achievement in the social realm a new form of relating to this power must be discovered. Yet this turning is also a returning, a return to the original source, a kind of homecoming.

The theme of homecoming pervaded my entire journey. To be open to place meant more to me than being susceptible to the power of self-evidently sacred space; I wanted also to be open to the lived significance of apparently profane spaces. I wanted to visit not only the museumized places restored and preserved by westerners (like the Taj Mahal or the Khajaraho temples) but the streets, houses, shops, bars that constituted the everyday world of the native residents. I wanted exposure to places that were loved, were home, were the center of the world to someone as my home was to me. Paradoxically, part of the point of my journey had become understanding better what it really means to be at home at home—a lesson Hölderlin suggests we are always taught by the wanderer.

There were teachers along the way who helped impress on me the full meaning of at-home-ness. Among them were two young men met in India who were radically *not* at home. One we met in Fatipuhr Sakri, a former Moghul capital not far from Agra but even older. The site is now a ghost town and was almost deserted while we were there. We spent several hours with a young student of architecture from London, Ghanian-born but of Indian descent, for whom visiting in India was proving hard. Many of the particulars of what made him uncomfortable—with the people, the climate, the cities, the customs—were those voiced by

Naipaul in the book in which he recounts his similar "return" to the land of his ancestors. To be shown the *pain* of this disillusioning exploration of the supposed "roots" was very sad—as was, paradoxically, to sense how much at home he felt with us. We'd come by crowded public bus, he by train, but he decided to go back with us. The press to get on the late and already crowded bus was, as so often, a tumultuous scene. Tom had football-shouldered his way onto the bus; I hadn't made my way *in* but had a secure foot on the steps and a good handhold on the outside bar and was confident of inching my way in after a stop or two. But our new friend literally pulled me off and said in horror, "Chris, Chris, you can't get on with those animals." So Tom somehow made his way out again and we all went back by train.

The other meeting occurred in Khajaraho. We were at the temples during those lovely golden late afternoon hours when India is at its most beautiful. There were no other tourists, so we had the fascinating temples and the beautifully planned expansive green gardens within which they are set to ourselves. Somehow we ended up being led around from temple to temple by a thirtyish man who spoke excellent English and seemed familiar with every carving inside and outside of every temple. A self-taught local villager who had grown up in their shadow, he clearly loved his surroundings *and* longed to be living a very different life somewhere else. He helped us see in a way we couldn't have on our own, for he knew the myths that underlay each sculpted scene and appreciated the craftsmanship that made some exceptionally powerful. Ingeniously, delightfully, he would pull us to yet another favorite—"This is the *most* beautiful." He seemed especially to enjoy showing us the most explicitly fantastic sexual scenes, and it was clear that all the scenes of threesomes were stirring his own fantasies.

He was a delightful guide, and knew enough to let us enjoy the last half hour of sunset in the gardens by ourselves. The next day we met him again quite by chance as we happened to walk by his door in one of the nearby villages. There in his own home as we sipped the tea he proudly served us and listened to his accounts of village life, it became even more evident to us how not at home he was. Though he had never been more than a few kilometers away from his birthplace, he was a radically unhomed human being.

Perhaps I was especially attuned to this because during the entire trip I was more radically cut off from any contact with my home than ever before in my life: with a companion from whom I was often painfully estranged, eating entirely unfamiliar food day after day, surrounded by people speaking languages I could neither use nor understand. The entire period in the Orient had the disorienting and reorienting impact traditionally associated with the liminal phase of passage ritual. I was indeed in another world, symbolically speaking in the other world. In India, more clearly than elsewhere, I experienced how different the world view and presuppositions of the inhabitants were from my own. I felt distance both from them and from my own familiar world. Indians seem to have little tolerance for small talk and a different sense than ours of what constitutes an intrusion of privacy or an invasion of personal space. Within a very few moments of beginning a conversation, I would be asked if I believed in God, how much money I made, whether I enjoyed sex, whether I approved of Indira and/or Reagan. Almost as immediately my interlocutors would be telling me about their vasectomies, their struggles to break free of the extended family, the disadvantages of arranged marriages, their ambitions for their children, their sense that most of India's difficulties were due to the Hindus or Muslims (whichever they weren't).

There seemed to be very little confidence that things were going to get much better for India as a whole, though often much hope that they themselves would be able to manipulate the sys-

tem to their own advantage. Familial loyalty seemed to be a
highly important value (though in a time of radical cultural transition it also provoked a lot of conflict and pain), but honesty in
an abstract sense seemed almost meaningless, as did any commitment to the well-being of the society as a whole. Their time
sense felt so different from mine — either very short-run or eter-
nal, with very little appreciation of "historical" time, the kind of
time required for significant social change. In India more emphatically than elsewhere I realized this trip had, indeed, taken
me "out of time" and into a mode of consciousness where prog-
ress, social achievement, and social roles were relativized as never
before. Not that I am done with them, but only that I now
somehow see through them.

Customarily the most important of the "fabulous forces" met
in the "region of supernatural wonder" are the men and women
who appear as teachers, whether as helpers or as hinderers. Traditionally, there are guides for such journeys. On our group tour
of China we were provided with guides in the most conventional
sense — guides who did not help us at all. But elsewhere I met
four men in their seventies the beauty of whose way of living old
age moved me deeply. They communicated that quality of fully
being themselves and knowing how to let that flow out to others
that I sense Freud had, and Jung too, and Buber. Of course, I
fell a little in love with each of them.

The first of these was our host in Tokyo, a Catholic priest,
who had lived in Japan almost all his adult life. He had survived
several heart attacks and major heart surgery; during our visit he
had several dream encounters with Death which he trusted me
to help him understand. He modeled an enthusiastic embrace
of life which included a reverent equanimity in the face of
death.

Second was Raavi, an Indian in whose village home we stayed
for several days. Smaller than I, widowed for many years, white-

haired, wracked by a terrible cough, Raavi may be the most intensely, passionately alive human being I have ever known. A small but faithful readership has allowed him to support his extensive extended family by the modern Hindi parables and speculative fiction which he's been writing for fifty years. Raavi is fascinated by utopian experiments and particularly by alternative life-styles. He has a wonderfully unconventional imagination and is acutely aware of the painful human cost of many traditional Hindu life patterns. (Not that he doesn't clearly and quite unself-consciously enjoy playing the patriarch. It is clear *everyone* is at his beck and call; but clear, too, that his daughters-in-law have a much easier time than if there were also a matriarch to deal with.) He was so fascinated by Tom and me that when he learned of the age difference between us and that I'd been married before and had children, he immediately created his own version of Tom's and my love affair which included a fantastically elaborated account of Tom stealing me from my husband. He kept telling us how inspiring Indians would find our willingness to follow the pull of romantic love. No matter how hard we tried to superimpose our own version, he preferred his own.

The third such encounter also occurred in India. Waiting for the train in Fatipuhr Sakri, I experienced one of those "only in India" scenes. A striking old, white-haired, white-bearded sadhu came up to me and began singing—partly in Bengali, partly in English—one of those Song of Songs kind of hymns where the erotic and the spiritual are inextricably intertwined. As his song went on and on, he and I looked unflinchingly at one another. A crowd gathered. "Thank you," he said. "I feel you are a very wise woman. Perhaps if you gave me your address, we could stay in touch." "No," I said, "I feel it is better to leave it like this. It feels complete to me. Neither of us will forget." He nodded his head in quiet agreement. When he had gone, one of the bystanders said, "You must be an important person in your country—that is a very holy man."

The fourth was an Australian physician, again in his seventies, whom I met on the long bus ride from the India-Nepal border to Katmandu: Once a world-famous surgeon, now, in "retirement," head of the largest hospital in Nepal, he spends most of his time trying to secure pure water for the villages and encouraging reforestation. While holding a sick child whom someone who knew absolutely nothing about him had nonetheless dumped in his lap and left there for the entire bus ride, he shared with me his contagious hopes for the future of Nepal where today forty percent of the children still die before they are five. He was, quite simply, a *radiant* human being.

These men are each very different, but I believe each has learned with utter modesty to make himself a *channel*. My exploration of goddess traditions had been initiated by a dream in which a wise old man appeared to proffer me his help. I brushed his offer aside as I told him that he and I had been through this before and that it was now time for me to go in search of "Her." Perhaps had I stayed at home to live through the menopausal transition, it would have been older women who would have appeared as my initiators. Yet for this trip these men, as gentle and compassionate as any woman, served as fitting complements to my young hero-companion, suggesting that there might be some truth after all to the image of old age as a phase of life where literal gender matters less and less. The female guides appeared after my return to help with the integration phase.

When I name the people met along the way teachers, that doesn't mean that even now I could tell you what I learned from them. I only know they entered deep into my soul; that I am somehow different because of our meeting, that in their presence I felt loved, re-energized, redirected. The meeting that I remember most vividly of all was entirely speechless:

On the long train journey from Singapore to Bangkok I sat for several hours face to face with two Malaysian prisoners, handcuffed to one another. One of their guards sat next to me; several others were across the aisle. Because no one spoke any English, my understanding of the situation is mostly conjecture. One of the prisoners was a very young, somehow simple-looking man who seemed bewildered and frightened. "How did my life get me here? This isn't how it was supposed to turn out." My sense was that the charges and punishment the two faced were very serious, that their crime probably had a political dimension. The other man was older, in his thirties, very intense and handsome. He and I spent a lot of time looking very directly and intently at one another, wondering and accepting. I was moved by the way this older man used the way the two were handcuffed together as an opportunity to keep his hand reassuringly on the other's knee, thigh, forearm. He, too, was clearly frightened and yet in some way seemed to have accepted that, yes, this was precisely what his life had brought him to.

Much of the time one of the guards (also very handsome, very quiet, very present) sat on the arm of their seat in a way that made it seem natural for him to have his arm around the older prisoner's shoulders and to communicate with innumerable gestures as well as with the tone and rhythm of his words his sympathy and his human concern. There was something very beautiful in these various gestures of male-male support. Toward the end of the afternoon, one of the women who had been sitting further back in the car came forward and wordlessly brought a little snack, rolls of curried rice wrapped in banana leaves, to the prisoners. As a real completion of these unforgettable hours, the older prisoner gave one to me.

THE ULTIMATE BOON

*This is the place of the break-through
into abundance.*

—Joseph Campbell

T hat the journey was unidirectional, bringing us home
without our ever having to turn around, did not mean
that there was no central climactic or paradigmatic
moment. There was for each of us.

The climax of the trip for Tom happened in Nepal just before
he was ready to fly to Europe and thus consciously turn homeward. He had been trekking alone in the Himalayas, and found
himself at the peak of his ascent with a magnificent view of Mach-
repachre, a mountain sacred to the Nepalese who believe that if
it were ever climbed, that would be the end of life in Nepal. So
the ascent has never been attempted. The discovery of a mountain that may not be climbed — what a perfect culmination of
the heroic quest, a deep and beautiful lesson.

The climax for me occurred in Bali, as it happened almost ex-
actly at the midpoint of the trip both spatially and temporally.
By then Bali had already impressed me as an island where the
mundane and the sacred are complexly interfused. Like almost
every other visitor to Bali I was impressed by the natural unself-
conscious spirituality of the culture. The living religiosity of Bali
was evident even in Kuta, the tourist-filled village which was
our base. There were household altars everywhere and many
temples. Every morning and night each threshold and each altar
was adorned with carefully constructed offerings of flower and

fruit, fragrant with incense. Many times each week there were processions through town—gorgeously dressed women, men, and children, gaily colored umbrellas, elaborate pyramids of fruits and flowers piled on heads, percussion bands with typically Indonesian instruments. The processions led to the beach or to one of the temples and culminated in rituals which included dance, mime, music, silence. There were also special ritual dance performances in villages throughout the island. Tom and I climbed a sacred volcanic mountain from which we could look across to Mt. Agung, which is to the Balinese what Delphi is to the Greeks. Though I had never heard of this place I recognized immediately that the magnificent, still active volcano looming above the lovely crater lake was, indeed, the navel of the world.

Yet my own most sacred moments during the time spent on Bali were not so much stirred by the Balinese beliefs and ceremonies, by *their* religiosity, as by my own response to the same physical environment, the same spiritual presences perhaps, which had inspired those rituals originally. The "breakthrough into abundance" which I experienced in Bali might seemingly have happened anywhere, anytime, without my ever even leaving home, but happened here at the midpoint of our journey.

One evening in Kuta I lay on my bed alone after having eaten a magic mushroom omelette for supper. What happened that night is on the surface something that could as easily have happened anywhere, anytime. It brought vividly back to mind an evening in Santa Cruz seven years earlier when I felt I discovered that there *is* a center to the center (*and* that I had never believed it to be so). This evening in Bali felt like the counterpart to that one, in intensity and in significance. During that night I relived many of the most important meetings of my life—some just as they had happened, others changed so as to actualize their latent or potential fullness—and lived also moments that haven't happened yet but may, or that could have happened at some earlier time but didn't and yet in some sense still can. The usual sense of temporal linearity seemed entirely dissolved—*it*, not this co-presence, seemed illusion. I felt surrounded (though in a way that permitted the full honoring of each) by the many I have loved or almost loved and the many who have loved me. I felt their very real presence. But much more important than the details was an overwhelming feeling of being loved enough.

I remembered how during the preceding summer I had been able (with a Gestalt therapist's quiet sure encouragement) to cry out for the fullness of love for which I have yearned all my life —and feeling then, there is a fulfillment in wholly experiencing the longing even when one is adult enough to accept that it won't ever be fully assuaged. A friend who was with me said that it seemed as though the harsh sounds that forced their way past my throat were the cries of a mother in labor, the cries of a new-born child.

What I felt that night in Kuta—and still feel—what I knew and know is that I *am* given enough love—enough to fill—and (as at Santa Cruz) that I never before truly believed that possible. I had such a vivid image that night of a whole circle of my friends standing around me, beaming at me and yet also teasing a little, as they said in chorus, "She's finally catching on." I had a vision of my turning to each of them and saying quite simply, "Thank you for having loved me enough."

No perilous task accomplished. No terrifying ordeal overcome. Simply a gift received in gratitude. Simply birth, rebirth.

THE CROSSING OF THE RETURN THRESHOLD

All seems familiar, even the hastening
greeting
Seems the greeting of friends, each
face seems congenial.
To be sure! It is the nativeland, the
soil of the homeland,
That which thou seekest is near and
already coming to meet thee.

The trip made me newly aware of the relativity of the sacred and the profane. As I set out, the strange lands to which my journey would take me appeared filled with numinosity; being on the journey made me aware of the holiness of home.

Certainly that the journey was to be a circular one whose goal all along was home had from the outset felt enormously important to me. Yet I had not fully realized then nor during the journey itself that the homecoming phase needed as much honoring as the more exotic earlier parts of the trip.

Though when we first set out we were none too sure we would ever make our way back, of course we did, though significantly, not together. The return, as is often true in the socially defined passage rites, took place in stages, thus enabling the reintegra-

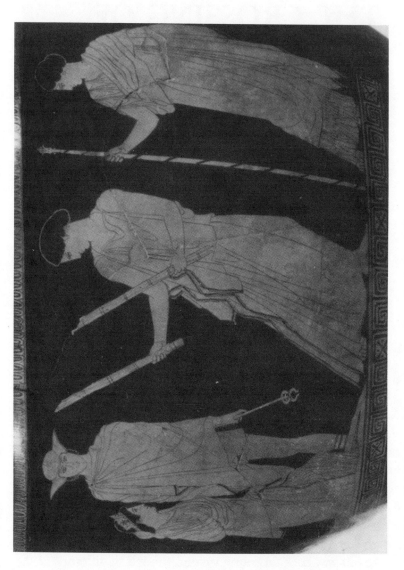

11. Hekate Lighting Persephone's Emergence from the Underworld, red-figured bell krater, Metropolitan Museum, New York.

tion itself to be a stage entire and not just a moment. Leaving India meant beginning the reentry phase — again a threshold sprinkled with blood and water. When my plane touched ground in Paris, I felt my cheeks wet with tears. I had not known to expect them. . . .

On that flight I had wakened with a pinched nerve that affected me painfully for the rest of the trip and for weeks after I returned. It was during the weeks spent in Europe that I first became aware of experiencing the "hot flashes" that so often accompany menopause. Perhaps I'd had them earlier but in the tropics not recognized them for what they were. No one had prepared me for how sensual this suffusion of one's body with internally generated heat could be. Whenever the hot flashes appeared in the months after my return, I welcomed them as a reminder, as physiological symbol, of all that had happened to me in the torrid zones through which the trip had taken us.

To be in Europe was to be in a different world; my unsettledness in Paris felt like a counterpart to the night of dreams in Seattle as we set out. The two realities, India and France, seemed as incommensurate as dream and waking — but it seemed impossible to settle on which was which. I'm not sure how well I would have handled having to cope with finding bed, food, entertainment in the overwhelmingly rich Parisian environment. Luckily, I was spared that by being able to stay a few days with the friend of a friend who lived in a quiet, elegant suburb. I did little but sleep, take walks in the grounds of the local chateau, and talk to my hostess, the first woman I'd been close to for months.

Yet though Europe was so radically different from Asia, I was soon reminded that I *was* still traveling. I laughed at some of the ways in which traveling in Europe seemed not all that different from traveling in India after all. Due to some equipment failure the train I'd planned to take from Paris to Basel had been canceled, so I had to go on a roundabout route via Strasbourg. Then when I finally got to Basel I discovered there was not a hotel room available in the city. Changing my just-acquired Swiss francs to German marks, I went on to Freiburg, despite my son's having advised me of the importance of starting the search for a room in always crowded Freiburg early in the day. But luck was with me and I did find a room. The price seemed appalling for a small (though clean and quiet) room without a bath: one night cost more than half of what I'd spent on lodging during our entire time in India and Nepal. My son's affirmation next day that I had done very well and his easy acceptance of what seemed to me the exorbitant cost of food and of train fare helped me begin to come to terms with the radically different financial scale.

Germany, my childhood home and a country I'd often stayed in as an adult, was more unfamiliar than I had expected. I was surprised at how radically Germany had changed since we lived in Tübingen in 1968. Then Germany had seemed comfortably shabby, the pace of everyday life and of cultural change had seemed slower than in America. Despite the horror of all they had lived through the Germans my own age seemed somehow more innocent or more naive than I, their children more so than mine. Just those ways in which Germany felt different from America were what made me feel at home there, as though the land of my birth was more in tune with my rhythms than the one I lived in most of my life. Now Germany seemed more prosperous, more modern, more busy, more self-satisfied — more American in a way — than America. Yet when the shops closed, when the streets emptied, the lovely old buildings, the cobbled pavements, and woods and hills immediately accessible from the very heart of the city in which one can walk in solitude for hours served as talismans of some still enduring stabilizing pattern of life.

I spent most of the week before Tom rejoined me with my son in Göttingen. Being with him felt like a preliminary homecoming as did finally getting some news of family. He could assure me that my parents were well, that my former husband seemed happy and centered in his new marriage, and brought me up to date on what each of his siblings was up to. When Tom arrived from Nepal, we spent a few weeks together in Scandinavia "debriefing," and then separated again. During a good part of our time together in Europe, Tom appeared to be in the throes of an overwhelming exhaustion, as though his body in its way were saying, "I've had enough." Clearly even when he was physically stronger, this seemed true for his soul. The Himalayas had, or so it felt as he spoke of them, touched him at his very core and filled him. There really was no room for any new experience. The Norwegian fjords were beautiful, Bergen a charming city, but somehow that seemed almost beside the point.

It seemed entirely appropriate for us *not* to return to California together. I flew straight home; he stopped in New York to visit his family. Thus the return journey was one each of us essentially made on our own. Homecoming had a very different meaning in his life than in mine. I was at a phase of my life where I *had* a home to return to, whereas Tom would be returning to the task of finding and making one. During the trip I became more conscious than I had been before of how important it was to have a home, not my parent's home or one I shared with husband and children but my own. In a way that had never before been true, "homecoming" meant not quest but simply return. I knew now as I had not earlier that there is for me a *here* from which the world discloses itself. I had discovered that traveling is different when one has such a here, that one enters other places differently. It allows one to see what a place means both to those who belong there and to you. It enables one to expose oneself fully to the experience of a new place and delight in what that place is doing to one, knowing that one's relation to it is different from that of those for whom it is home.

A few days after my arrival in California, I wrote: "And now I am home, ready to be here, though not quite knowing yet what that means." I had returned a few days earlier than scheduled and found I did not want to let anyone know of my premature arrival. It felt important to live those first days of homecoming as a solitary experience. We had bought our tickets on the winter solstice; I returned just prior to the summer solstice. To celebrate my return and the year's turning I went to the sacred mountain near the Mexican border that has for years been for me a place of integration and discovery. I knew I could not yet articulate how the returning self was different from the one who had left and yet nevertheless wanted to symbolize the fact of a change by adopting a new name, "Christine" (as at the time I entered adolescence, "Tini" had become "Chris"). I knew I had returned as a postmenopausal woman. I felt myself more fully identified with my womanly self than ever before: ready to write my sisters book, ready to make relationships with women central. I felt I had come home ready to stay put, to be a more settled person (in my soul, not simply outwardly, literally) than ever before. I felt I had discovered the sacrality of home and that the trip had in large measure been directed to that discovery: "Whoever passes through the various positions of a lifetime one day sees the sacred where before he has seen the profane."[24] I truly knew that I am loved enough.

IV
THE RETURN

COMING HOME TO HESTIA

She bore
none of her usual attributes;
the Child was not with her . . .
she wasn't hieractic, she wasn't frozen
she wasn't very tall;
she is the vestal
from the days of Numa,
she carries over the cult
of the Bona Dea,
she carries a book but it is not
the tome of the ancient wisdom,
the pages, I imagine, are the blank
  pages
of the unwritten volume of the new . . .
This is no rune nor symbol,
what I mean is — it is so simple
yet no trick of the pen or brush
could capture that impression;
what I wanted to indicate was
a new phase, a new distinction of
  colour.

—H.D.

131

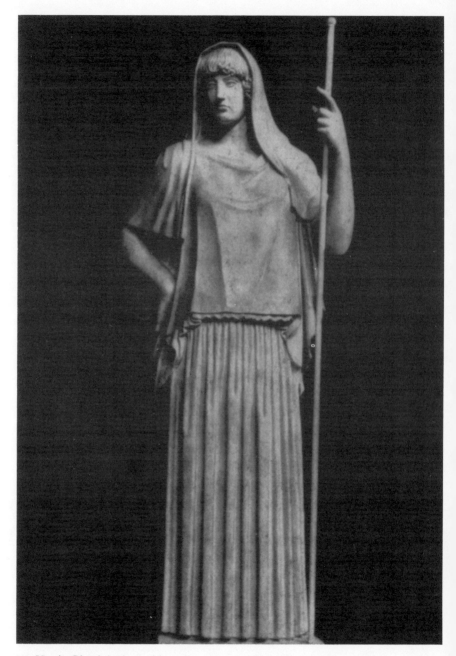

12. Hestia Giustiniani, marble, 5th c. B.C.E., Villa Albani, Rome.

Before even beginning my preparation for menopause I had given honor to each of the great goddesses of ancient Greece: to Demeter, Hera, Athene, Aphrodite, and Artemis. I knew that together with Zeus, Poseidon, Apollo, Hermes, Ares, Hephaistos, and Dionysos they were represented on the east frieze of the Parthenon as constituting the canonical divine family, "The Twelve," whose cult was founded by Herakles and by whom the Greeks were wont to swear. I understood Persephone's and Hades' conspicuous absence from this pantheon as attributable to their being underworld divinities, not denizens of Olympos nor concerned with the daily oath-provoking occasions "The Twelve" might help one with. And, in any case, I had given them their due.

But, then, without warning, after my return from my trip around the world a thirteenth divinity stepped forth to claim her place: Hestia, the goddess of the hearth and home. Her appearance was as unexpected as that of the thirteenth fairy who comes without invitation to Briar Rose's christening celebration. Of course, I had known that some versions of The Twelve included Hestia, but the discrepancy had never seemed of any great interest to me nor had she herself assumed any importance in my life — until my return from that journey whose hidden destination seems all along to have been this homecoming. In many ways, I had never really *seen* her. The Greeks knew Hestia was owed the first and last offering. My homage is a belated one. May it suffice.

My former neglect of Hestia bespeaks not so much conscious avoidance or denial as an unattending taking for granted. I remember how surprised I was to learn that there are almost no Earth signs in my astrological chart. That seemed disconsonant with my own sense of myself and with my teacher's. "Maybe," she said, "that is because your relation to Earth is not a task for this lifetime; perhaps it has already been accomplished." What our lives rest on may be most invisible. She also told me that having Cancer in the ascendent points to a capacity for homelife which becomes most significant in old age and directed me toward Hexagram 57 of the *I Ching*, "The Gentle," the hexagram of the eldest daughter. Casually she noted how the preceding hexagram speaks of "The Wanderer" who "has nothing that might receive him; hence there follows the hexagram of the gentle, the penetrating. The gentle means going into, homecoming."[1] The chart was cast years before my wandering or my homecoming.

On coming home I began to understand that to miss Hestia is to miss the feminine in what may be its most essential aspect: that is, how easily it is invisible, ignored, disvalued and yet *there* as the presupposition of all else — sustaining even when not noticed, not demanding attention, not going after us, but immediately available when we return to her. Hestia is not present in the extraordinary as are the other goddesses but in the midst of the most ordinary and mundane. Plato's playful derivation of her name from *ousia*, essence, communicates her essentiality; his observation that "Hestia alone abides at home" expresses her hiddenness and continual availability.

Since Hestia is the goddess of the home and the hearth, it is not surprising that I only discover her divinity upon returning home. I see now that my journey was all along a journey toward her, a coming back, as T. S. Eliot puts it, to the place from which I started and knowing it for the first time. The journey toward Hestia is not a journey toward a luminous unknown but toward the luminous known, toward the discovery of the holiness of the most familiar. Hestia represents that strange fusion of the *heimlich* and the *unheimlich* (literally, the home-like and the un-home-like) which Freud analyzes in his essay on "The Uncanny." *Heimlich* means not only the familiar, friendly, intimate, but that which is concealed, secret, withheld, that which is obscure, inaccessible to knowledge, unconscious: it is closely related to *Geheimnis*, secret. "Heimlich is a word the meaning of which develops toward an ambivalence, until it finally coincides with its opposite, *unheimlich* (the uncanny or mysterious). *Unheimlich* is in some way or other a subspecies of *heimlich* . . . The *unheimlich* is what was once *heimlich*, home-like, familiar; the prefix 'un' is the token of repression." The "uncanny is in reality nothing new or foreign but something familiar and old-established in the mind that has been estranged," something which has been kept concealed but nevertheless comes to light.[2] Freud helps me see in Hestia the hidden holiness of that which is most familiar coming to illumination.

I discovered this holiness only on *returning* home, but perhaps Hestia is always discovered thus. In his lecture on Hölderlin, "Remembrance of the Poet," Heidegger suggests that the recognition that proximity to the source is a mystery is only open to the returning wanderer. Homecoming is the discovery that the holy is near, that it is present in "the gentle spell of well-known things and the simple relations they bear to one another" —and at the same time remains reserved, at a distance, remains mystery. The innermost essence of home, he writes, is the hearth of the house which is the source of serenity, of joy, of healing. Though Hölderlin believes that "holy names are lacking," that simply to say "Hestia" does not enable us at home to be at home, nevertheless to call her name is to bring her near.

Heidegger understands that home means more than "a house and the merely casual possession of domestic things." Hestia makes a house a home by endowing it with soul. It is her gift to reveal how my dwelling serves as an outward expression of my inward self and how the image of the inmost center of a dwelling, its hearth, serves as the most adequate, the almost inevitable, image of the essence of self.[3] Though soul and psyche are not physically locatable, we seem to need spatial language to speak of them; they appear to us as "inner" realities. I sense Hestia's presence in my house, especially in the intimately enclosed area in front of the living-room fireplace. I also sense her presence in the secret underground chamber accessible only to me of my earliest remembered dreams. The name Hestia helps me to recognize the homology between these two experiences of sacred space.

When I first returned from my journey, however, her name did not occur to me. I knew I was now, in ways mostly still to be discovered, a different person, as one is after participating in any rite of passage. It seemed apt that I had come back just in time to celebrate the summer solstice, just at that time of year when the days begin to grow shorter. The world to which I returned was familiar—and strange. The life I had left when I set out felt too big for me to reoccupy it, and too cluttered. I came home physically thinner, but it was not only my clothes that hung loose, that didn't quite fit; my very being had somehow been concentrated, simplified. It was to mark the change that I decided that I, who since puberty had always preferred to be called Chris, was now Christine. Although I still felt ambivalent about the "pristine" associations this name provoked for me, I knew it was time to claim the more feminine and more mature way of being in the world it represented.

In some way I had become her—Christine—was no longer in quest of her. This was a time for assimilation, integration rather than search, a time for staying put, for dwelling with. Halfway through my journey I had had the profound mystical experience, the vision in which I found myself surrounded by those who love me and knew, "I am loved enough." I had always believed that my yearning for love was insatiable but now found that I was full. I was ready to come home then, and also ready to undertake the months of traveling that still lay between me and home. Now at home I hoped to discover how real that fullness was and how it might shape my everyday life.

The goddesses I had invoked to help prepare me for meno-pause no longer seemed particularly pertinent. Hekate's super-vision of transition, Rhea's modeling of grandmotherly devo-tion, Baubo's exuberant delight in her own sexuality seemed irrelevant to the work, the home-work, to which I now felt call-ed. At first it appeared that what I now needed to do was to at-tend to the ordinary, the everyday, that I had moved into a period when I would no longer be actively engaged with *any* of the goddesses. I presumed a correlation between the divine and the extraordinary and thought of myself as back in Auden's "for the time being":

> Back in the moderate Aristotelian city
> of darning and the Six-Fifteen, where Euclid's geometry
> And Newton's mechanics would account for our experience,
> And the kitchen table exists because I scrub it.

Sometimes content, sometimes aware (as Auden's narrator also is) that:

> The Time Being is, in a sense, the most trying time of all.[4]

At first it did not even occur to me that holiness might be found in the ordinary, the safe, the repetitive, the anonymous.

Until I read Kathryn Rabuzzi's *The Sacred and the Feminine*[5] I had not remembered that the Greeks had seen divinity in this homely aspect of feminine energy and named it Hestia. I then immediately recognized Hestia as goddess of the third phase of the traditional pattern of the rite of passage, the phase of return, incorporation, where, as Joseph Campell puts it, "all is enjoyed and known unconsciously in the space 'within the heart.'" She represents what he refers to as "the ultimate state of anonymous presence," "the revelation of a plenum of silence within and around every atom of existence."[6]

But to continue to see the holiness of the most mundane and familiar, to keep Hestia in sight, proved difficult. The flame on the hearth flickers and disappears. I feel drawn to her and antagonized. What she asks—to see the numinous in the everyday, the trivial—is so simple, and therefore so hard. Sometimes her realm seems luminously, simply beautiful; at other moments unbearably boring. In *such* moments it is easy, indeed to understand how easily she lost her place among The Twelve or why the Roman near-equivalent, Vesta, was made into a much grander and more visibly powerful goddess. It is also painful to glimpse that serenity, that joy of being at home at home of which Hölderlin writes, and then to feel it slip away.

Among the Greeks Hestia's blessing was invoked not only at every festival but at the simplest household meal: she was worshiped not at some specially designated temple but at the family hearth. She is the thirteenth Olympian: one comes to her *after* one has paid homage to all others. It seems appropriate that in at least some parts of Greece her attendants were elderly once-married women. Though ageless like all goddesses, there is something middle-aged about Hestia who is so essentially "beyond" marriage and childbearing and something about her more likely to appeal to us in our own later years.

To acknowledge Hestia is to relate to all the other goddesses differently. Allegiance to her does not conflict with one's devotion to any of them, although it tempers it. Hestia received the first and last offering at every feast, no matter what divinity was being honored. Hestia teaches modesty, humility, moderation. She puts in question the illusions of the Great Quest, the Great Love, the Great Struggle, the Great Insight, the Great Renunciation, the Great Solitude.

Prosaic, concrete, iconoclastic, she creates suspicion of the extraordinary, of all that we usually mean by divine. Again I think of Auden:

How can his knowledge protect his desire for truth from illusion?
   How can he wait without idols to worship, without
Their overwhelming persuasion that somewhere, over the high hill,
   Under the roots of the oak, in the depths of the sea,
Is a womb or a tomb wherein he may halt to express some attainment?
   How can he hope and not dream that his solitude
Shall disclose a vibrating flame at last and entrust him forever
   With its magic secret of how to extemporize life?[7]

As H. D. sees, in Hestia's light things do not function as rune or symbol; "it is so simple" — a new phase, a new distinction of color.

We bring our experience to Hestia for illumination, assimilation, integration. Things fall into place, assume their proper proportion; complicated connections, elaborate amplifications, abstruse interpretations seem beside the point. We, too, are put in our place. The distinctive quality of Hestian illumination is integrally related to her being goddess of the hearth. In his *Psychoanalysis of Fire* Gaston Bachelard offers a description of Hestia-inspired reverie:

> The fire confined to the fireplace was no doubt for man the first object of reverie, the symbol of repose, the invitation to repose.... It leads to a very special kind of attention which has nothing in common with the attention involved in watching or observing. Very rarely is it utilized for any other kind of contemplation. When near the fire, one must be seated: one must rest without sleeping; one must engage in reverie on a specific object.... This reverie is entirely different from the dream by the very fact that it is always more or less centered upon one object. The dream proceeds on its way in a linear fashion, forgetting its original path as it hastens along. The reverie works into a star pattern. It returns to its center to shoot out new beams.[8]

As I wrestled to understand and accept Hestia, I saw how important it is that she is not the only goddess. Seen in isolation she would demand passivity rather than what I take to be the *work* of this life phase: bringing the other divinities home, putting their gifts and curses in perspective. I had sensed during my journey that it was time for me to move beyond the emphasis on the distinctive qualities of each of the highly differentiated goddesses of the Greek pantheon and to move towards an integration of feminine energies that might have the full power of the original undifferentiated mother goddesses. In India Kali had appeared as a symbol of such reintegration. At home that radically different figure, Hestia, came forward in Kali's place. Not alone but with her sisters.

In the fairytale, as P. L. Travers observes, "The Thirteenth Wise Woman becomes the Wicked Fairy solely for the purposes of one particular story. It was by chance that she received no invitation: it might just as well have been one of her sisters."9 But it is no chance matter that Hestia is the thirteenth Olympian. There is something integral to her essential being that occasions it. She was one of the original Olympians, sister to Demeter and Hera, and to Hades, Poseidon, and Zeus, indeed the firstborn of Kronos' and Rhea's children, but according to tradition, when late-arriving Dionysos appeared she modestly gave up her place among The Twelve to him. A tradition but no story. (As we shall see, it is somehow typical of Hestia that there should be no story.) All we know is that on the Akropolis frieze overlooking Dionysos' theatre, he has a place among the Olympians, she does not.

My suspicion is that the canonical Twelve represent a fiction, like the fiction that there are twelve tribes of Israel, as there are twelve signs of the zodiac. The imposition of the fiction may be related to the attempt to reconcile the solar and lunar calendars, may be sign of the triumph of the patriarchal solar perspective.

A matriarchal moon-centered calendar has thirteen months and for a goddess-centered perspective thirteen is a lucky number. Hestia as the thirteenth divinity may represent all that is suppressed when this perspective is lost. When she is replaced by a male god, the balance between masculine and feminine energies within the Pantheon is lost, and until we recover a sense of her, the cost of that loss has not been fully acknowledged. The thirteenth goddess is the first—rediscovered. Hölderlin writes of "the time when god's failure helps."[10] Hestia's absence, when experienced *as* absence, may also help.

Hestia's apparent invisibility, her anonymity and impersonality, are related to her being an unstoried, plotless goddess. Homer ignores her because there are no stories to tell, which may help explain my own neglect as well. Hestia requires a reconsideration of my preference for myth over archetype, narrative over image, and of the degree to which this prejudice represents a devaluation of some prototypically feminine reality. She puts in question my proclivity for storytelling. Making stories of my dreams and my adventures betrays as well as honors, conceals as much as it reveals. The stories may lead away from the inner center, the source of illumination and growth-nurturing warmth. To sacrifice to Hestia is something that is done in private, secretly; it is an intimate family ritual to which no outsiders are admitted. I do not mean that story as such is a masculine mode; heroic quest does not exhaust the meaning of story. Demeter's search, Persephone's abduction, Ariadne's giving guidance and subsequently being abandoned, Hera's jealous struggles, Aphrodite's wooing of Anchises, Artemis' deadly rejection of Actaeus, Athene's inadvertent slaying of her childhood playmate, Pallas—all these are stories whose plots differ significantly from the traditional curve of the hero's story. Nor are these simply stories men tell about women to demean them; they are tales women tell about themselves—even if in the received versions we can often discern the imprint of a patriarchally inspired re-telling.

Hestia's unstoriedness exists in the context of her storied sisters, just as Artemis's wildness and solitariness are given their meaning by contrast with the social imbeddedness of the other Olympian goddesses. As Artemis is not the primordial nature goddess but the goddess who deliberately shuns the civilized world, so Hestia, who refuses any response to her would-be suitors, Apollo and Poseidon, is the goddess who deliberately avoids entanglement and adventure. That Hestia never leaves Olympos or her hearth reminds us that plot means place before it means narrative.[11]

Hestia may remind us of that aspect of the feminine which is hidden, disvalued, and often self-demeaning, but she also offers a subtly powerful critique of our tendency to define ourselves in ego terms, by reference to our outward accomplishments and visible successes.

Hestia represents a denigrated aspect of the feminine. In this she is both like and unlike her sister Hera. Unlike, because Hestia is not explicitly devalued by the classical Greek authors, precisely because there are almost *no* stories, no Homeric references, and so few literary allusions. She, much more truly than Athene, is the goddess about whom no unworthy tales are told. Her darkness is the darkness of obscurity, not of evil or ugliness. (She is not "homely" in that sense.) Her hiddenness is not an artifact of patriarchal repression but integral to her, consonant with what we learn of her from cultic tradition. Though she is the last goddess I came to reckon with, she is the oldest of all the Olympians, in some sense the representative among them of the pre-Olympian world. Though displaced from the official roster of The Twelve, she is in no way a peripheral goddess: her place is at the very center of Olympos, of the polis, of the familial home, of the soul. To pay due homage to her demands recognition of that centrality, involves rediscovery of the fullness of what it means to be Hestia, both the creative and the destructive element, and of her uniqueness.

This least anthropomorphic of the Olympian deities evokes an earlier period of animistic belief. Farnell suggests that this may be due to her name continuing to serve as a common noun designating the hearth or its fire, just as "Gaia" continued to mean simply the earth: "As the name 'hearth' clung to her, she could not emerge and develop into a free personality with an individual and complex character or history, like Artemis or Athena." Yet he also observes that "there is no trait in her that reveals a glimpse of a prehistoric nature-goddess or elemental daimon."[12] Unlike Gaia, Hestia retains no chthonic primordial energies. Though a goddess of place she has no apparent relation to fertility or to the underworld; rather she is associated with place in its most domesticated aspect, with the center of the family home or of the polis. Like the other Olympians she is closely related to the human sphere. As navel of the earth, the omphalos at Delphi was originally associated with Gaia; as the sacred fire tended by the Pythia, it is Hestia's. When the oracle is taken over by Apollo and recognized as the place for Greeks to bring their most pressing personal and political concerns, Hestia becomes the goddess "who takes care of the holy house of Apollo" with "a liquid oil flowing forever from [her] hair."[13]

Hestia's impersonality thus has a very different meaning from Gaia's; it receives its significance within a personal and interpersonal context. I see her—this goddess who is invoked both first and last—as pertaining to human selfhood both in its predifferentiated beginnings and in its reach toward ego-transcendence. I see her also as having to do with an interconnection between human beings that consists simply of a quiet acceptance of one another, free of any attempt to impress or change, of any need to possess or reject.

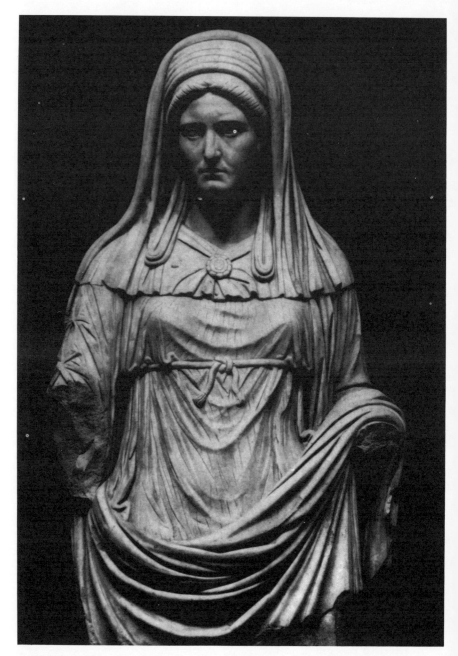

13. Vestal, marble, Roman period, Museo Nazionale della Terme, Rome.

The first literary reference to Hestia as a personal goddess is found in Hesiod's *Theogony* where she is spoken of as the oldest daughter of Rhea and Kronos, the first to be swallowed by her usurpation-fearing father and the last to be disgorged when Zeus appears to liberate his siblings. Hestia is the goddess imprisoned longest in the patriarchal womb and thus the one who may appear to have most lost the primal potency of the archaic goddesses and to have the least individual character. Hestia's impersonality and her anonymity seem to bear a double meaning, to have an original significance *and* an imposed one. The enforced passivity serves to blind us to an original quiescence which has quite a different meaning. We are likely to see in Hestia a representation of the repressed feminine as itself an archetypal reality. We see her as embodying impotence, a fear or incapability of self-assertion, rather than a mode of divine power.

Especially in her Roman form, as Vesta, she is associated with a pre-personal femininity. In Rome she was served by virginal attendants chosen before they were six years old, swallowed as Hestia had been so early they could not yet have achieved any individual character. But in Greece she seems also to represent a post-personal femininity; at Delphi she was served by an elderly once-married woman who no longer lived with her husband. The double vision is one I cannot seem to overcome; at times I see her as robbed of her individuality, at times as having transcended it. The dominant Greek understanding is clearly that her way of being is chosen, integral, not an external imposition. She is honored by the offering of a *willing* sacrifice: the ox that spontaneously bows its head is the one dedicated to Hestia.[14]

Seeing her in relation to the other Olympian goddesses helps us to see her more clearly, though we need to remember that she is related to them in an uneventful non-narrative mode — as a distinct image, a particular essence. Hestia never actively differentiates herself; she simply is. The Greeks rarely represented Hestia in anthropomorphic form in their statues, bas reliefs, or pottery, nor are there any attributes which clearly mark a figure as hers. Statues which are explicitly identified as portraying Hestia show her with scepter and with veil—a perfect rendering of the hiddenness of her power. Yet no less than any of the other goddesses does Hestia "shape and illumine the whole compass of human existence with [her] peculiar spirit."[15]

Both Demeter and Hera share Hestia's long childhood immersion in their father's belly but each responds distinctively to the common infantile experience. Certainly it did not issue in deep bonding among them; Demeter and Hera were perceived as so intrinsically opposed to one another that when the temple of one was open, the temple of the other would be closed; there are no traditions about either ever interacting with Hestia. All three, each radically deprived of infantile mothering, become mother goddesses—though in contrast with Gaia their mothering is domesticated and defined by the male dominance of the world they were born into.

Though Demeter is goddess of the grain, she is associated primarily with domestic agriculture. What is most distinctive about her is her intense devotion to her daughter, Persephone— a devotion which seeks to protect Persephone from any contact, paternal or sexual, with the world of men. Hestia's mothering is more peculiar: "The child was not with her." She is a mother without children of her own (as in a sense was true of her mother before her). She is a virginal goddess who in sculpture is portrayed with the large full breasts of the nursing mother. She is mother to the unmothered; Alcestis calls on Hestia to protect her soon-to-be-orphaned children. In Rome, Vesta by virtue of the unpossessiveness of her maternal care, comes to be regarded as the epitome of the ideal mother. Yet to that part of me which insists on seeing Hestia in negative terms, her childlessness represents sterility. On the other hand, as a mother with literally no children, with no literal child, Hestia represents a feminine generativity that transcends biological mothering. This, too, makes her a goddess particularly relevant to postmenopausal women. When I wrote my book about the Greek goddesses, I ended it with a meditation on the child as image of the still unfolding self. Hestia both seems to represent what it means to be related to such a soul-child and to suggest that she herself, the thirteenth divinity, comes forward as a different, after-the-more-obvious goddesses, self-image. Hestia is not only pre-Olympian but post-Olympian, the goddess beyond the goddesses.

Hera is essentially wife, the woman who continues to look to the masculine for nurturance and her own completion, who struggles against patriarchal privilege and is defined by that struggle. Her children are simply pawns in that primary engagement with her spouse, Zeus. Hestia is housewife without ever being wife, devoted not to spouse *or* child but to the family as such. She explicitly begs Zeus to free her from the obligation to marry. Her dispassionate, non-possessive protectiveness may strike us as beautiful, or as expressive of a pathological fear of intimacy. Sometimes we may feel that she stayed in Kronos too long.

At other times, even more than Athene or Artemis, Hestia seems to embody the essence of virginity, of in-one-selfness, of a mode of feminine being not defined by any relationship. The Homeric Hymn to Aphrodite speaks of Hestia as:

> The lady that
> Poseidon and Apollo were both after. She
> didn't want them, she refused them firmly.
> and she swore a great oath on it, one that
> was fulfilled, touching the head of father
> Zeus who carries the aegis, that she would
> be a virgin every day, a divine goddess.[16]

Hestia's immunity to Aphrodite may well be the aspect of her with which I have the greatest difficulty. Aphrodite, too, represents an in-one-selfness in relationship. Hers is an unpossessed and unpossessing love, a love that belongs to the moment and makes no claims on the future. Aphrodite's love is centrifugal, it flows out from her. Hestia's love is centripetal, it pulls us home. Her love has a quality of utter trustworthiness, conveys continuity and stability. Hestia seems to play no favorites; she loves whoever comes to her hearth; the direction of her loving is not determined by fantasy or feeling. Where Aphrodite embodies spontaneity as truth, Hestia signifies even-flowing commitment, staying power. She binds the new to the old. The newly married daughter's hearth is lit with a burning log brought from her mother's household, and so it has been since time immemorial.

It is important clearly to distinguish Hestia from the other two goddesses exempt from Aphrodite's lures, from Artemis and from Athene. Hestia's virginity, never at threat, never needing defense, is even more primordial than that of Artemis. Her essential self-containment is achieved simply by staying where she is; there is no necessity to flee to the wilderness. She exhibits none of the passionate self-assertion implicit in Artemis' choice of solitude and celibacy. Her privacy is of a different kind and can be maintained even in company. The radical quality of Artemis' claims is utterly foreign to Hestia. The extravagant self-sacrifice of the Roman Vestal virgins is, I am coming to believe, a subtle betrayal of what Hestia really asks, which is the sacrifice even of sacrifice writ large.

Like the other virginal goddess, Athene, Hestia nurtures communal (as well as familial) ties. Though, except at Elis, there were no temples in Greece specifically designated as hers, there was an altar to her in the center of the council chambers of every Greek city, a communal hearth. The establishment of a colony was symbolized by bringing a log from the mother city's hearth to the new city's central hall. In Rome the Palladium, symbol of the city's inviolability, was kept in Vesta's temple. Hestia is a protectress of the polis though not engaged as Athene is in its active defense. She has nothing to do with the heroic or the adventuring spirit. Athene actively accompanies and supports the wandering home-seeking Odysseus; Hestia is present with patiently waiting, stay-at-home Penelope. (Though like Penelope, Hestia welcomes the returning wanderer.) Penelope's weaving, unweaving, reweaving is an excellent image of the repetitive, unchanging, undramatic constancy of Hestian devotion. Both Athene and Hestia have a practical, moderating, reality-principle dimension; but where Athene relies on her quickness of mind, her inventiveness, and her resolute courage, Hestia makes do with what is and recognizes the need for compromise, for accommodation.

A Euripidean fragment identifies Hestia with yet another virgin, Persephone. Both are goddesses associated with a particular place: Persephone with the underworld, the inside of the earth; Hestia with the hearth, the inmost part of the house. Etymology suggests an intimate connection between Hestia's sphere and the realm of the dead: Our word "home" derives from the Indo-European root *kei* (to lie, bed, night's lodging, home, beloved) by way of the Germanic *hiwa; kei* reappears unchanged in Greek and in a variant form, *koiman*, which means put to sleep, is the origin of our word "cemetery."[17] The Vestal temples were round like the ancient Greek tombs; the most important Vestalian ritual was celebrated in the spring at the beginning of the New Year when the sacred fire in the Roman temple was rekindled. Thus Hestia, like Persephone, is a soul goddess, but in her realm soul-experience is not associated with an afterworld but as something available in the midst of the everyday. Even death is somehow not a "big deal"; the family's life continues, the hearth stays lit. Nor does Hestian consciousness initiate us into a recognition of the symbolic significance of everyday things or events. "There is no rune or symbol." There is no especial initiation into Hestia's cult at all: Farnell even maintains that there is no mention of Hestia in connection with the Amphidromia, the ritual in which a five-day-old infant is carried around the hearth and given its name. The connection to Hestia is always already there.

Fully to understand Hestia requires that we look also at her relation to the male divinities. That Apollo and Poseidon are both would-be suitors suggests that a relation to her is in some way essential to them, whereas her indifference to their proposals indicates she has no need of them. Perhaps Apollo's cool rationality would benefit from contact with her gentle warmth and down-to-earthness; perhaps Poseidon's association with the turbulent ocean depths seeks the complement of her quiet, drying heat. It may be, however, that the tradition of the marriage offers is merely a playful explanation of the joint worship of the three divinities at Delphi, an instance of myth following rite.

The connection to Zeus is of more obvious significance. He is both younger brother and rescuer. Hestia, never really taken in by his claims of machismo power, neither serves him nor has to fight against him. Only she does not participate in the attempted revolt against him when the other Olympians surround him as he lies asleep and tie him to his bed. The implicit equality between them is suggested by a bas-relief which shows Zeus with Hestia at his side in Hera's usual place, both being waited upon by Ganymede. Hestia's place is not only at the center of home and city but at the center of Olympos itself. As Plato says, in the dwelling of the gods, Hestia alone abides at home. The most famous statue of her among the ancients was that at Scopas which portrays her seated, immobile. She is thus the central figure of

the Greek pantheon, though her hegemony has an entirely different character than Zeus'. She isn't hieratic (or hierarchical);
she isn't frozen; she isn't very tall. She seems to have no need to
insist on her priority and unlike Zeus does not seem to live in
fear of its being jeopardized. She receives the first libation at every sacrifice but seems unperturbed that greater attention is paid
to the subsequent offerings to the other deities. Still, "to sacrifice to Hestia" *means* to give completely; no part of the offering
may be taken away or given to others.

Zeus overshadows Hestia only by almost being her. It is Zeus
of the hearth, Zeus *Ephestios*, who is the personal divinity invoked as the central figure not only in the city cult but even in
the domestic one. Libations are offered to the Hestian Zeus; her
altars, other than the hearth itself, become his. For Hestia is
most adequately represented simply by the hearth fire itself.
The paucity of sculptural representations is due to the recognition that the right way to imagine her presence is as the fire, not
in personal form.

There seems to be no point of contact between Hestia's cult
and the cult of the other Greek fire deity, Hephaistos. His temples stand outside the city walls; her place is at the city's very
center. His is the fire of smith and potter and of the volcano,
hers the smoldering coals of the domestic hearth. His is the fire
of technology and art, hers the fire of ritual which may not go
out. In her realm fire is more a social than a natural reality. Bachelard tells us that "what we first learn about fire is that we must
not touch it." Hestia's fire is thus a virginal fire, fire become a
symbol of purity, of sublimation, a fire which totally consumes
that which it burns. Her controlled fire becomes an image of
sublimation as a joyful activity, a joyful acceptance of limitations. "The haphazard passion becomes the deliberate passion.
Love becomes family; fire becomes hearth and home." In

Hestia's realm passion may be made luminous without being cooled, love pure and ardent at once.[18] Cook notes that the Pythagorean Hestia is the equivalent of the Platonic Ananke;[19] Hestia teaches that same acceptance of necessity, limitation, finitude Freud saw as the essence of maturity.

As we have seen, Bachelard believes that "the first use and the truly human use of fire" is the reverie it encourages:

> We are almost certain that fire is precisely the first object, the *first phenomenon,* on which the human mind reflected; among all phenomena, fire alone is sufficiently prized by prehistoric man to wake in him the desire for knowledge, and this mainly because it accompanies the desire for love. No doubt it has been stated that the conquest of fire definitely separated man from the animal, but perhaps it has not been noticed that the mind in its primitive state, together with its poetry and its knowledge, has been developed in meditation before a fire.... The *dreaming man* seated before his fireplace is the man concerned with inner depths, a man in the process of development. Or perhaps it would be better to say the fire gives to the man concerned with inner depths the lesson of an inner essence which is in a process of development.[20]

Though the sacrificial fire is Hestia's, she does not become the primary mediator between earth and heaven as Agni does in the Vedic tradition. Hers is specifically the fire that makes home home. She is a divinely immanent power from whom we learn the immanence, the indwelling, of the divine.

Although Hestia is absent from the Parthenon's relief, she is paired with Hermes in many of the archaistic reliefs of The Twelve. There are also many ancient double-faced (Janus-form) busts in which Hestia and Hermes are joined, looking in opposite directions. These two divinities are linked also in one of the Homeric Hymns to Hestia:

> And you too, Argeiphontes, son of Zeus and Mala,
> messenger of the gods, with your golden wand,
> giver of good things, be good to me,
> protect me along with the venerable and dear Hestia.
> Come, both of you inhabit this beautiful house
> with mutual feelings of friendship.[21]

Their association is not explicable simply on the basis of the tradition that Hermes was the inventor of kindling fire. Though Hermes is the phallos that stands at the entry to every house, their pairing is not sexual; in Hestia's presence Hermes represents familial fertility. She abides at the center of the house, he stands at the threshold, marking the boundary between inside and outside, blessing all departure and returns. Both signify a clear sense of boundaries, of the difference between in and out. Hestia stays herself, she is in no danger of merging with lover or spouse or child. Hestia stays the same; Hermes is a shapeshifting god, associated with movement, change, transformation. Hestia stays at home: Hermes is the wayfaring, message-bearing god. Their frequent pairing expresses these complementaries.

Both deities symbolize beginnings: Hestia as firstborn of the Olympians, Hermes as the childlike, playful, tricky. Hermes is often invoked as the god of depth psychology; he is psychopomp and interpreter. James Hillman writes that depth psychology looks:

> for its truths in error in which deeper, more central necessities lie . . . Hermes, who cheats his father Zeus as soon as he is born, is the congenital deceiver bringing equivoca-

tion into the world with divine authority. He is god of equivocation as he is guide of the soul. And we each sense him when we would speak most deeply of our souls, for just then we feel the error, the half-truth, the deception in what we are telling.... No one can tell the real truth, the whole truth about the soul but Hermes whose style is that of duplicity.[22]

But Hestia, too, is a soul-guide, one whose way is not interpretation but illumination, reflection, focus, a simple staying with that which appears. Her impersonality, her silence, remind me of Freud's sense of how *therapaia* is most effectively accomplished: she heals by *not* responding. She gives so little — and so much.

The Olympian who most helps us see what it means to come home to Hestia is, however, that other god of going and coming, appearing and disappearing, Dionysos. That he can replace her among The Twelve suggests that he represents an even more essential complement: The god who is neither recognized nor acknowledged in his own home, Thebes, is also the god who easily succeeds in inveigling stuck-at-home housewives into frenzied participation in his mountaintop orgies. More radically than Hermes, Dionysos is the god of the border. Life in his realm has meaning *at* the edge, at the limit, at the extreme; Hestia remains goddess of the center. To look at him and then at her is to be forced to ask: Is it better to be crazy or bored? Is meaning found in ecstasy or the everyday? To stay with these questions — as Hestia would invite us to do — is to begin to understand why she voluntarily relinquishes her place to him and still is as much at home on Olympos as ever. Hestia is no Pentheus, she does not deny Dionysian reality; she is never his antagonist.

"Hestia alone *abides* at home" — it is so easy to misunderstand, to see her as demanding we do the same. I struggle with how difficult it is for me, even now, even past menopause, to stay with a perspective that pays homage to the holy in The Ordinary, The Boring, The Everyday. I laugh as I realize how unHestian that challenge is. My homework for this new phase of my life is to acknowledge the holy in the ordinary, the boring, the everyday.

My journey through menopause has brought me to Hestia. She comes bearing none of the usual attributes of the goddess but carrying a book with blank pages, the unwritten volume of the new. I am only beginning to sense what will be written there.

NOTES

I. PREAMBLE

1. Arnold Van Gennep, *The Rites of Passage* (Chicago: University of Chicago Press, 1950), pp. 189f., 194.
2. Mircea Eliade, *Rites and Symbols of Initiation* (New York: Harper & Row, 1965), pp. 128, 135.
3. Erik Erikson, *Childhood and Society* (New York: W. W. Norton & Co., 1953), p. 270.
4. Quoted in Simone de Beauvoir, *The Coming of Age* (New York: G. P. Putnam's Sons, 1972), p. 4.
5. Jane Rule, "Grandmothers," *Outlander* (New York: Persephone Press, 1981), p. 207.
6. C. G. Jung, "The Stages of Life," *The Collected Works*, vol. 8 (New York: Pantheon, 1960), p. 399.
7. C. G. Jung, *Memories, Dreams, Reflections* (New York: Pantheon, 1963), pp. 170–99.
8. Eliade, *Rites*, p. 41ff. Eliade says "sign" not symbol; the transposition on my part is deliberate. I am following Paul Tillich in distinguishing "signs" as arbitrary, conventional substitutions from "symbols" which participate in that which they signify.
9. Eliade, *Rites*, pp. 42, 47.
10. Cf. Valerie Saiving Goldstein, "Androcentrism in Religious Studies," unpublished mss.
11. Cf. Nancy A. Falk and Rita M. Gross, eds., *Unspoken Worlds: Women's Religious Lives in Non-Western Cultures* (San Francisco: Harper & Row, 1980).
12. Van Gennep, *Rites*, p. 145.
13. De Beauvoir, *Age*, p. 2.
14. Adrienne Rich, *The Dream of a Common Language* (New York: W. W. Norton, 1978), p. 70.
15. Cf. Madeleine Goodman, "Toward a Biology of Menopause," in Catherine R. Stimpson and Ethel Spector Pearson, *Women: Sex and Sexuality* (Chicago: University of Chicago Press, 1980), p. 253.
16. M. Esther Harding, *The Way of All Women* (New York: Harper & Row, 1973), pp. 245ff.

17. Goodman, "Biology," p. 264; Marilyn Grossman and Pauline B. Bart, "Taking the Men Out of Menopause," in Ruth Hubbard, Mary Sue Henifin, and Barbara Fried, eds., *Women Look at Biology Looking at Women* (Cambridge, MA: Schenkman, 1979), pp. 163–86.

18. Audre Lorde, *The Cancer Journals* (Argyle, NY: Spinsters, Ink, 1980), p. 9.

19. Van Gennep, *Rites*, p. 192. (His italics.)

II. PREPARATION

1. Paula Weidegger, *Menstruation and Menopause* (New York: Alfred A. Knopf, 1976), p. 44.

2. Simone de Beauvoir, *The Second Sex* (New York: Bantam Books, 1961), p. 541.

3. C. G. Jung and C. Kerenyi, *Essays on a Science of Mythology* (Princeton, NJ: Princeton University Press, 1969), p. 101. Kerenyi has borrowed the quotation from Frobenius's *Der kopf als Schicksal*.

4. Helene Deutsch, *The Psychology of Women*, vol. 2: *Motherhood* (New York: Bantam Books, 1973), pp. 476–509 passim.

5. De Beauvoir, *The Second Sex*, p. 541.

6. Deutsch, *The Psychology of Women*, vol. 2, p. 481.

7. Weidegger, *Menstruation and Menopause*, pp. 161–63.

8. De Beauvoir, *The Second Sex*, p. 28.

9. Mary Daly, *Gyn/Ecology* (Boston: Beacon Press, 1978), p. 248.

10. Maurice R. Green, ed., *Interpersonal Psychoanalysis: The Selected Papers of Clara M. Thompson* (New York: Basic Books, 1964), p. 279.

11. De Beauvoir, *The Second Sex*, p. 542.

12. Cf. Weidegger, *Menstruation and Menopause*, p. 45.

13. Cf. Robert M. Stein, "Body and Psyche," *Spring*, 1967, p. 67.

14. Donald J. Dalessio, *Migraine* (West Orange, NJ: Organon, n.d.), p. 1.

15. Daly, *Gyn/Ecology*, pp. 16, 15.

16. L. R. Farnell, *The Cults of the Greek States*, vol. 2 (Chicago: Aegaean Press, 1971), p. 510.

17. Erwin Rohde, *Psyche* (New York: Harper & Row, 1966), pp. 297ff. and passim.

18. M. Esther Harding, *The Way of All Women* (New York: Harper & Row, 1975), pp. 254f.

19. Irene Claremont de Castillejo, *Knowing Woman* (New York: Harper & Row, 1973), p. 157.

20. Deutsch, *The Psychology of Women*, vol. 2, p. 478.

21. David Bakan, *And They Took Themselves Wives* (San Francisco: Harper & Row, 1979), pp. 24, 118, 122.

22. Gerhard von Rad, *Genesis* (Philadelphia: Westminster Press, 1961), p. 238.

23. Deutsch, *The Psychology of Women*, vol. 2, p. 504.

24. Cf. David L. Miller, "Red Riding Hood and Grand Mother Rhea," in James Hillman, ed., *Facing the Gods* (Dallas: Spring Publications, 1980), pp. 87–100.

25. Deutsch, *The Psychology of Women*, vol. 2, p. 496. To be fair to Deutsch I should acknowledge that she, too, sees that some of the long-buried interests of youth may be revived at menopause, that energy long tied up in the productivity of motherhood may now be released for intellectual and artistic creation. For her, too, there may be a positive aspect to the postmenopausal woman's identification with her prepubertal self. Cf. p. 478.

26. Cf. James Hillman, "Puer and Senex," in Hillman, ed., *Puer Papers* (Dallas: Spring Publications, 1979), pp. 3–53.

27. Jung and Kerenyi, *Essays on a Science of Mythology*, p. 101.

28. De Beauvoir, *The Second Sex*, p. 281.

29. Barbara Myerhoff, "The Older Woman as Androgyne," *Parabola* 3, no. 4 (November 1978): 75.

30. Cf. June Singer, *Androgyny* (New York: Anchor Press, 1977), esp. p. 314.

31. Cf. C. Robert May, *Sex and Fantasy* (New York: W. W. Norton,

1980), p. 173; and Margaret Mead, *Male and Female* (New York: New American Library, 1955), p. 275.

32. Ovid, *Metamorphoses*, trans. Mary M. Innes (Baltimore: Penguin Books, 1955), pp. 102–4. In the text it says Diana, not Artemis.

33. Deutsch, *The Psychology of Women*, vol. 2, pp. 482–84.

34. Deutsch, *The Psychology of Women*, vol. 2, pp. 485f.

35. Harding, *The Way of All Women*, p. 252.

36. Deutsch, *The Psychology of Women*, vol. 2, p. 494.

37. Russell A. Lockhart, "Cancer in Myth and Disease," *Spring*, 1977, p. 2.

38. Thomas Mann, *The Black Swan* (New York: Alfred A Knopf, 1971), p. 140.

III. THE PASSAGE

1. Arnold Van Gennep, *The Rites of Passage* (Chicago: University of Chicago Press, 1960), pp. 11, 191.

2. Elizabeth Bishop, *The Complete Poems 1927–1979* (New York: Farrar, Straus, Giroux, 1983), p. 94.

3. Paul Fussell, *Abroad: British Literary Traveling Between the Wars* (New York: Oxford University Press, 1980), p. 37.

4. Joseph Campbell, *The Hero with a Thousand Faces*, (New York: Meridian Books, 1956), p. 97.

5. Carl Kerenyi, *Zeus and Hera* (Princeton: Princeton University Press, 1975), p. 5.

6. By Mark Schorer as quoted in Fussell, p. 143.

7. May Sarton, *Collected Poems 1930–1973* (New York: W. W. Norton, 1974), p. 244.

8. Quoted in E. Relph, *Place and Placelessness* (London: Pion Limited, 1976), p. 10.

9. Quoted in Fussell, *Abroad*, p. 209.

10. Campbell, *The Hero*, p. 30.

11. Van Gennep, *Rites*, p. 194.

12. Donald R. Howard, *Writers and Pilgrims: Medieval Pilgrimage Narratives and Their Posterity* (Berkeley: University of California Press, 1980), frontispiece. (Of course Odysseus's journey, too, was a home-directed one but he is represented as the prototypical *anti*-hero who relies on trickery not bravery and chooses survival over glory.)

13. Mircea Eliade, *Rites and Symbols of Initiation* (New York: Harper & Row, 1965), p. 136.

14. Fussell, *Abroad*, p. 43.

15. Robert Scholes and Robert Kellogg, *The Nature of Narrative* (New York: Oxford University Press, 1966), p. 73.

16. Cf. Lonnie D. Kliever, "Story and Space: The Forgotten Dimension," *Journal of the American Academy of Religion* 45/2 Supplement (June 1977), G:579–613.

17. Margaret Atwood, *You Are Happy* (New York: Harper & Row, 1974), p. 75f.

18. Quoted in Fussell, *Abroad*, p. 117ff.

19. Van Gennep, *Rites*, p. 18.

20. Rainer Maria Rilke, "Orpheus/Eurydice/Hermes" in Stephen Mitchell, editor and translator, *The Selected Poetry of Rainer Maria Rilke* (New York: Random House, 1982), pp. 51, 53.

21. Victor W. Turner, *Image and Pilgrimage in Christian Culture* (New York: Columbia University Press, 1978), p. 13.

22. Cf. Annis Pratt, *Archetypal Patterns in Women's Fiction* (Bloomington: Indiana University Press, 1981), chs. 6, 8, 9.

23. Sarton, *Collected Poems*, p. 236f.

24. Van Gennep, *Rites*, p. 13.

IV. THE RETURN

1. Richard Wilhelm and Cary F. Baynes, translators, *The I Ching* (Princeton: Princeton University Press, 1967), p. 679.

2. Sigmund Freud, "The Uncanny," *Studies in Parapsychology* (New York: Collier Books, 1963), pp. 30, 51, 47.

3. Martin Heidegger, "Remembrance of the Poet," *Existence and Being* (Chicago: Henry Regnery Company, 1949), pp. 243–70.

4. W. H. Auden, "For the Time Being," *Collected Poems* (New York: Random House, 1976), pp. 307–8.

5. Kathryn Allen Rabuzzi, *The Sacred and the Feminine: Toward a Theology of Housework* (New York: The Seabury Press, 1983). Cf. also Barbara Black Koltuv, "Hestia/Vestia," *Quadrant* 10, no. 2 (Winter 1977): 57–65; Stephanie A. Demetrakopoulos, "Hestia, Goddess of the Hearth," *Spring*, 1978, pp. 55–76; Barbara Kirksey in James Hillman, ed., *Facing the Gods* (Irving, Texas: Spring Publications, 1980), pp. 101–13.

6. Joseph Campbell, *The Hero with a Thousand Faces* (New York: Meridian Books, 1956), pp. 266, 237, 267.

7. Auden, "For the Time Being," *Poems*, p. 275.

8. Gaston Bachelard, *Psychoanalysis of Fire* (Boston: Beacon Press, 1964), pp. 14, 15 (slightly rearranged).

9. P. L. Travers, *About the Sleeping Beauty* (New York: McGraw-Hill, 1975), p. 56.

10. Heidegger, "Remembrance," p. 265.

11. Cf. Lonnie D. Kliever, "Story and Space: The Forgotten Dimension," *Journal of the American Academy of Religion* 45/2 Supplement (June 1977), G:579–613.

12. Lewis Richard Farnell, *The Cults of the Greek States* (Chicago: Aegean Press, 1971), pp. 364, 357.

13. Charles Boer, translator, *The Homeric Hymns* (Chicago: Swallow Press, 1970), p. 141.

14. Arthur Benard Cook, *Zeus*, III, 1 (Cambridge, England: Cambridge University Press, 1940), p. 565.

15. Walter F. Otto, *The Homeric Gods* (Boston: Beacon Press, 1964), p. 160.

16. Boer, *Homeric Hymns*, p. 73.

17. *The American Heritage Dictionary of the English Language* (New York: American Heritage Publishing Co., 1969), s.v. "kei," p. 1521, in "Indo-European Roots."

18. Bachelard, *Fire*, pp. 11, 100, 101.

19. Cook, *Zeus*, II, p. 316.
20. Bachelard, *Fire*, pp. 14, 55f.
21. Boer, *Homeric Hymns*, p. 140.
22. James Hillman, *ReVisioning Psychology* (New York: Harper & Row, 1975), p. 160.

DATE DUE

GAYLORD   PRINTED IN U.S.A.